Also by Jonathan Bailor

The Smarter Science of Slim:
What the Actual Experts Have Proven About Weight Loss, Health, and Fitness

The Smarter Science of Slim Workbook:
The Five-Week Harvard Medical School, Johns Hopkins, and UCLA
Endorsed Program To Burn Fat Permanently

THE SMARTER SCIENCE OF SLIM JOURNAL

A Smarter Way to Track Your Weight Loss

Jonathan Bailor

Aavia Publishing
Fewer, better books™

New York • Seattle

Published in the United States, Canada, and the U.K. by Aavia Publishing. New York. Seattle. www.AaviaPublishing.com.

Aavia Publishing books can be purchased at quantity discounts to use as premiums, promotions, or for corporate training programs. For more information on bulk pricing please email Aavia Publishing at http://www.AaviaPublishing.com/contact.

Editor: Mary Rose Bailor
Interior Design: Adina Cucicov, Flamingo Designs
Exterior Design: Michael David McGuire
Cover Photo: Douglas Gorenstein

Special appreciation to Michael David McGuire and his media team in New York. McGuire's unique insights and guidance helped greatly strengthen this project.

Publisher's Cataloging-in-Publication

Bailor, Jonathan.
The Smarter Science of Slim Journal: A Smarter Way to Track Your Weight Loss / Jonathan Bailor.—1st ed.
p. cm.
ISBN 978-0-9835208-4-9
1. Health   2. Weight Loss   3. Physical Fitness   4. Exercise   5. Diet   6. Nutrition   7. Self-Help
I. Bailor, Jonathan II. Title.

Manufactured in the United States of America. First Edition.

Dedication

To you and everyone else with the courage to eat and exercise smarter. You have taken the road less traveled and it will make all the difference.

Week 1—Day 1   Date: Mon June 3

		Ate:	Target:
Non-Starchy Vegetables	Ate: Target:	□□□□□□□□□□□ ■■■■■■■■■■■	
Seafood/Lean Meat/Egg Whites/Whey/Select Dairy	Ate: Target:	☑☑☑□□□□□□□□ ■■■■■	
Flax Seeds/Nuts	Ate: Target:	☑☑☑□□□□□□□□ ■■■■■	
Berries/Citrus Fruits 2C blueberries	Ate: Target:	☑☑☑☑□□□□□□□ ■■■■■	
Legumes	Ate: Target:	□□□□□□□□□□□	
Other Fruits	Ate: Target:	□□□□□□□□□□□	
Most Dairy	Ate: Target:	□□□□□□□□□□□	
Fatty Meat/Oils	Ate: Target:	□□□□□□□□□□□	
Starchy Vegetables/Starch	Ate: Target:	□□□□□□□□□□□	
Sweets/Sweetened Drinks	Ate: Target:	□□□□□□□□□□□	

Today I am proud that I: _____

_____

_____

Today I noticed that eating more and exercising less—smarter—
had a positive impact on my life when: _____

_____

_____

_____

What I ate today: _____
_____
_____
_____
_____
_____
_____
_____
_____
_____

What did I do well? _____
_____
_____
_____
_____
_____
_____
_____
_____
_____

Tomorrow I can eat more—smarter—5% more effectively by:
_____
_____
_____
_____
_____
_____
_____
_____
_____

Week 1—Day 2   Date:

Non-Starchy Vegetables	Ate:	☐☐☐☐☐☐☐☐☐☐
	Target:	■■■■■■■■■■
Seafood/Lean Meat/Egg Whites/Whey/Select Dairy	Ate:	☐☐☐☐☐☐☐☐☐☐
	Target:	■■■■■
Flax Seeds/Nuts	Ate:	☐☐☐☐☐☐☐☐☐☐
	Target:	■■■■■
Berries/Citrus Fruits	Ate:	☐☐☐☐☐☐☐☐☐☐
	Target:	■■■■■
Legumes	Ate:	☐☐☐☐☐☐☐☐☐☐
	Target:	
Other Fruits	Ate:	☐☐☐☐☐☐☐☐☐☐
	Target:	
Most Dairy	Ate:	☐☐☐☐☐☐☐☐☐☐
	Target:	
Fatty Meat/Oils	Ate:	☐☐☐☐☐☐☐☐☐☐
	Target:	
Starchy Vegetables/Starch	Ate:	☐☐☐☐☐☐☐☐☐☐
	Target:	
Sweets/Sweetened Drinks	Ate:	☐☐☐☐☐☐☐☐☐☐
	Target:	

Today I am proud that I: _____

_____

_____

Today I noticed that eating more and exercising less—smarter—
had a positive impact on my life when: _____

_____

_____

_____

What I ate today: _____

_____

_____

_____

_____

_____

_____

_____

_____

What did I do well? _____

_____

_____

_____

_____

_____

_____

_____

_____

_____

Tomorrow I can eat more—smarter—5% more effectively by:

_____

_____

_____

_____

_____

_____

_____

_____

_____

Week 1—Day 3   Date:

Non-Starchy Vegetables	Ate:	☐☐☐☐☐☐☐☐☐☐☐
	Target:	■■■■■■■■■■■
Seafood/Lean Meat/Egg Whites/Whey/Select Dairy	Ate:	☐☐☐☐☐☐☐☐☐☐☐
	Target:	■■■■■
Flax Seeds/Nuts	Ate:	☐☐☐☐☐☐☐☐☐☐☐
	Target:	■■■■■
Berries/Citrus Fruits	Ate:	☐☐☐☐☐☐☐☐☐☐☐
	Target:	■■■■■
Legumes	Ate:	☐☐☐☐☐☐☐☐☐☐
	Target:	
Other Fruits	Ate:	☐☐☐☐☐☐☐☐☐☐
	Target:	
Most Dairy	Ate:	☐☐☐☐☐☐☐☐☐☐
	Target:	
Fatty Meat/Oils	Ate:	☐☐☐☐☐☐☐☐☐☐
	Target:	
Starchy Vegetables/Starch	Ate:	☐☐☐☐☐☐☐☐☐☐
	Target:	
Sweets/Sweetened Drinks	Ate:	☐☐☐☐☐☐☐☐☐☐
	Target:	

Today I am proud that I: _____

_____

_____

Today I noticed that eating more and exercising less—smarter—
had a positive impact on my life when: _____

_____

_____

_____

What I ate today: _____

_____

_____

_____

_____

_____

_____

_____

_____

_____

What did I do well? _____

_____

_____

_____

_____

_____

_____

_____

_____

_____

_____

Tomorrow I can eat more—smarter—5% more effectively by:

_____

_____

_____

_____

_____

_____

_____

_____

_____

_____

Week 1—Day 4   Date:

		Ate:	Target:
Non-Starchy Vegetables	Ate:	□□□□□□□□□□□	
	Target:	■■■■■■■■■■■	
Seafood/Lean Meat/Egg Whites/Whey/Select Dairy	Ate:	□□□□□□□□□□□	
	Target:	■■■■■	
Flax Seeds/Nuts	Ate:	□□□□□□□□□□□	
	Target:	■■■■■	
Berries/Citrus Fruits	Ate:	□□□□□□□□□□□	
	Target:	■■■■■	
Legumes	Ate:	□□□□□□□□□□	
	Target:		
Other Fruits	Ate:	□□□□□□□□□□	
	Target:		
Most Dairy	Ate:	□□□□□□□□□□	
	Target:		
Fatty Meat/Oils	Ate:	□□□□□□□□□□	
	Target:		
Starchy Vegetables/Starch	Ate:	□□□□□□□□□□	
	Target:		
Sweets/Sweetened Drinks	Ate:	□□□□□□□□□□	
	Target:		

Today I am proud that I: _____

_____

_____

Today I noticed that eating more and exercising less—smarter—had a positive impact on my life when: _____

_____

_____

_____

What I ate today: _____

_____

_____

_____

_____

_____

_____

_____

_____

What did I do well? _____

_____

_____

_____

_____

_____

_____

_____

_____

Tomorrow I can eat more—smarter—5% more effectively by:

_____

_____

_____

_____

_____

_____

_____

_____

Week 1—Day 5   Date:

Non-Starchy Vegetables	Ate:	☐☐☐☐☐☐☐☐☐☐
	Target:	■■■■■■■■■■
Seafood/Lean Meat/Egg Whites/Whey/Select Dairy	Ate:	☐☐☐☐☐☐☐☐☐☐
	Target:	■■■■■
Flax Seeds/Nuts	Ate:	☐☐☐☐☐☐☐☐☐☐
	Target:	■■■■■
Berries/Citrus Fruits	Ate:	☐☐☐☐☐☐☐☐☐☐
	Target:	■■■■■
Legumes	Ate:	☐☐☐☐☐☐☐☐☐☐
	Target:	
Other Fruits	Ate:	☐☐☐☐☐☐☐☐☐☐
	Target:	
Most Dairy	Ate:	☐☐☐☐☐☐☐☐☐☐
	Target:	
Fatty Meat/Oils	Ate:	☐☐☐☐☐☐☐☐☐☐
	Target:	
Starchy Vegetables/Starch	Ate:	☐☐☐☐☐☐☐☐☐☐
	Target:	
Sweets/Sweetened Drinks	Ate:	☐☐☐☐☐☐☐☐☐☐
	Target:	

Today I am proud that I: _____

_____

_____

Today I noticed that eating more and exercising less—smarter—had a positive impact on my life when: _____

_____

_____

_____

What I ate today: _____

_____

_____

_____

_____

_____

_____

_____

_____

_____

What did I do well? _____

_____

_____

_____

_____

_____

_____

_____

_____

_____

_____

Tomorrow I can eat more—smarter—5% more effectively by:

_____

_____

_____

_____

_____

_____

_____

_____

_____

Week 1—Day 6   Date:

		Ate:	Target:
Non-Starchy Vegetables	Ate:	□□□□□□□□□□□	
	Target:	■■■■■■■■■■	
Seafood/Lean Meat/Egg Whites/Whey/Select Dairy	Ate:	□□□□□□□□□□□	
	Target:	■■■■■■	
Flax Seeds/Nuts	Ate:	□□□□□□□□□□□	
	Target:	■■■■■	
Berries/Citrus Fruits	Ate:	□□□□□□□□□□□	
	Target:	■■■■■	
Legumes	Ate:	□□□□□□□□□□□	
	Target:		
Other Fruits	Ate:	□□□□□□□□□□□	
	Target:		
Most Dairy	Ate:	□□□□□□□□□□□	
	Target:		
Fatty Meat/Oils	Ate:	□□□□□□□□□□□	
	Target:		
Starchy Vegetables/Starch	Ate:	□□□□□□□□□□□	
	Target:		
Sweets/Sweetened Drinks	Ate:	□□□□□□□□□□□	
	Target:		

Today I am proud that I: _____

_____

_____

Today I noticed that eating more and exercising less—smarter—
had a positive impact on my life when: _____

_____

_____

_____

What I ate today: _____

_____

_____

_____

_____

_____

_____

_____

_____

_____

What did I do well? _____

_____

_____

_____

_____

_____

_____

_____

_____

_____

Tomorrow I can eat more—smarter—5% more effectively by:

_____

_____

_____

_____

_____

_____

_____

_____

_____

Week 1—Day 7 Date:

Non-Starchy Vegetables	Ate:	☐☐☐☐☐☐☐☐☐☐☐
	Target:	■■■■■■■■■■
Seafood/Lean Meat/Egg Whites/Whey/Select Dairy	Ate:	☐☐☐☐☐☐☐☐☐☐☐
	Target:	■■■■■
Flax Seeds/Nuts	Ate:	☐☐☐☐☐☐☐☐☐☐☐
	Target:	■■■■■
Berries/Citrus Fruits	Ate:	☐☐☐☐☐☐☐☐☐☐☐
	Target:	■■■■■
Legumes	Ate:	☐☐☐☐☐☐☐☐☐☐☐
	Target:	
Other Fruits	Ate:	☐☐☐☐☐☐☐☐☐☐
	Target:	
Most Dairy	Ate:	☐☐☐☐☐☐☐☐☐☐
	Target:	
Fatty Meat/Oils	Ate:	☐☐☐☐☐☐☐☐☐☐
	Target:	
Starchy Vegetables/Starch	Ate:	☐☐☐☐☐☐☐☐☐☐
	Target:	
Sweets/Sweetened Drinks	Ate:	☐☐☐☐☐☐☐☐☐☐
	Target:	

Today I am proud that I: _____

_____

_____

Today I noticed that eating more and exercising less—smarter— had a positive impact on my life when: _____

_____

_____

_____

What I ate today: _____
_____
_____
_____
_____
_____
_____
_____
_____
_____

What did I do well? _____
_____
_____
_____
_____
_____
_____
_____
_____
_____

Tomorrow I can eat more—smarter—5% more effectively by:
_____
_____
_____
_____
_____
_____
_____
_____
_____

Week 1 Eccentric Exercise

Date: *June 3 Mon*
5:30-6:30
to Katie

Home Option

		Add resistance?
Assisted Eccentric Squats	Resistance: _____	Y / N
Assisted Eccentric Pull-Ups	Resistance: _____	Y / N
Assisted Eccentric Push-Ups	Resistance: _____	Y / N
Assisted Eccentric Shoulder Press	Resistance: _____	Y / N

Gym Option

✱5min Bike Warmup Level 3
X6 Reps Each Side

		Add resistance?	
Total Gym Eccentric Leg Presses	*Rungs* Resistance: *R3 L8*	Y /(N)	*Knees*
Seated Row Eccentric Rows	Resistance: *30lbs*	(Y)/ N	*→35lbs*
Total Gym Eccentric Check Presses	Resistance: *2nd Rung*	Y /(N)	
Dumbbells Eccentric Shoulder Presses	Resistance: *R15 L12*	Y /(N)	

✱

Week 1 Cardiovascular Exercise

Date: *June 6 Thurs*

✱ 5min warm up
(30sec 2min Rest) X 6

		Add resistance?
10 Minutes of High-Quality Brief Cardiovascular Exercise	Resistance: _____	Y / N

✱ 5min cool down

Remember: *It should be impossible to do more than six repetitions of each eccentric exercise per week. It should also be impossible to do more than six repetitions of brief cardiovascular exercise per week. If more repetitions are possible or more workouts are possible, then add resistance.*

Notes: _____

_____

_____

_____

_____

_____

_____

_____

_____

_____

What did I do well? _____

_____

_____

_____

_____

_____

_____

_____

_____

_____

Next week I can exercise less—smarter—5% more effectively by:

_____

_____

_____

_____

_____

_____

_____

_____

Week 2—Day 1   Date:

Non-Starchy Vegetables
Ate: □□□□□□□□□□□
Target: ■■■■■■■■■■■

Seafood/Lean Meat/Egg Whites/Whey/Select Dairy
Ate: □□□□□□□□□□□
Target: ■■■■■

Flax Seeds/Nuts
Ate: □□□□□□□□□□□
Target: ■■■■■

Berries/Citrus Fruits
Ate: □□□□□□□□□□□
Target: ■■■■■

Legumes
Ate: □□□□□□□□□□□
Target:

Other Fruits
Ate: □□□□□□□□□□□
Target:

Most Dairy
Ate: □□□□□□□□□□□
Target:

Fatty Meat/Oils
Ate: □□□□□□□□□□□
Target:

Starchy Vegetables/Starch
Ate: □□□□□□□□□□□
Target:

Sweets/Sweetened Drinks
Ate: □□□□□□□□□□□
Target:

Today I am proud that I: _____
_____
_____

Today I noticed that eating more and exercising less—smarter—had a positive impact on my life when: _____
_____
_____
_____

What I ate today: _____

_____

_____

_____

_____

_____

_____

_____

_____

_____

_____

What did I do well? _____

_____

_____

_____

_____

_____

_____

_____

_____

_____

_____

Tomorrow I can eat more—smarter—5% more effectively by:

_____

_____

_____

_____

_____

_____

_____

_____

_____

_____

Week 2—Day 2   Date:

Non-Starchy Vegetables Ate: ☐☐☐☐☐☐☐☐☐☐☐☐
Target: ■■■■■■■■■■■

Seafood/Lean Meat/Egg Whites/Whey/Select Dairy Ate: ☐☐☐☐☐☐☐☐☐☐☐☐
Target: ■■■■■■

Flax Seeds/Nuts Ate: ☐☐☐☐☐☐☐☐☐☐☐☐
Target: ■■■■■■

Berries/Citrus Fruits Ate: ☐☐☐☐☐☐☐☐☐☐☐☐
Target: ■■■■■■

Legumes Ate: ☐☐☐☐☐☐☐☐☐☐☐☐
Target:

Other Fruits Ate: ☐☐☐☐☐☐☐☐☐☐☐☐
Target:

Most Dairy Ate: ☐☐☐☐☐☐☐☐☐☐☐☐
Target:

Fatty Meat/Oils Ate: ☐☐☐☐☐☐☐☐☐☐☐☐
Target:

Starchy Vegetables/Starch Ate: ☐☐☐☐☐☐☐☐☐☐☐☐
Target:

Sweets/Sweetened Drinks Ate: ☐☐☐☐☐☐☐☐☐☐☐☐
Target:

Today I am proud that I: _____
_____
_____

Today I noticed that eating more and exercising less—smarter—had a positive impact on my life when: _____
_____
_____
_____

What I ate today: _____

_____

_____

_____

_____

_____

_____

_____

_____

_____

What did I do well? _____

_____

_____

_____

_____

_____

_____

_____

_____

_____

Tomorrow I can eat more—smarter—5% more effectively by:

_____

_____

_____

_____

_____

_____

_____

_____

_____

Week 2—Day 3   Date:

Non-Starchy Vegetables	Ate:	☐☐☐☐☐☐☐☐☐☐
	Target:	■■■■■■■■■■
Seafood/Lean Meat/Egg Whites/Whey/Select Dairy	Ate:	☐☐☐☐☐☐☐☐☐☐
	Target:	■■■■■
Flax Seeds/Nuts	Ate:	☐☐☐☐☐☐☐☐☐☐
	Target:	■■■■■
Berries/Citrus Fruits	Ate:	☐☐☐☐☐☐☐☐☐☐
	Target:	■■■■■
Legumes	Ate:	☐☐☐☐☐☐☐☐☐☐
	Target:	
Other Fruits	Ate:	☐☐☐☐☐☐☐☐☐☐
	Target:	
Most Dairy	Ate:	☐☐☐☐☐☐☐☐☐☐
	Target:	
Fatty Meat/Oils	Ate:	☐☐☐☐☐☐☐☐☐☐
	Target:	
Starchy Vegetables/Starch	Ate:	☐☐☐☐☐☐☐☐☐☐
	Target:	
Sweets/Sweetened Drinks	Ate:	☐☐☐☐☐☐☐☐☐☐
	Target:	

Today I am proud that I: _____

_____

_____

Today I noticed that eating more and exercising less—smarter—
had a positive impact on my life when: _____

_____

_____

_____

What I ate today: _____
_____
_____
_____
_____
_____
_____
_____
_____
_____

What did I do well? _____
_____
_____
_____
_____
_____
_____
_____
_____
_____

Tomorrow I can eat more—smarter—5% more effectively by:
_____
_____
_____
_____
_____
_____
_____
_____
_____

Week 2—Day 4   Date:

		Ate / Target
Non-Starchy Vegetables	Ate:	☐☐☐☐☐☐☐☐☐☐☐
	Target:	■■■■■■■■■■
Seafood/Lean Meat/Egg Whites/Whey/Select Dairy	Ate:	☐☐☐☐☐☐☐☐☐☐☐
	Target:	■■■■■
Flax Seeds/Nuts	Ate:	☐☐☐☐☐☐☐☐☐☐☐
	Target:	■■■■■
Berries/Citrus Fruits	Ate:	☐☐☐☐☐☐☐☐☐☐☐
	Target:	■■■■■
Legumes	Ate:	☐☐☐☐☐☐☐☐☐☐
	Target:	
Other Fruits	Ate:	☐☐☐☐☐☐☐☐☐☐
	Target:	
Most Dairy	Ate:	☐☐☐☐☐☐☐☐☐☐
	Target:	
Fatty Meat/Oils	Ate:	☐☐☐☐☐☐☐☐☐☐
	Target:	
Starchy Vegetables/Starch	Ate:	☐☐☐☐☐☐☐☐☐☐
	Target:	
Sweets/Sweetened Drinks	Ate:	☐☐☐☐☐☐☐☐☐☐
	Target:	

Today I am proud that I: _____

_____

_____

Today I noticed that eating more and exercising less—smarter—
had a positive impact on my life when: _____

_____

_____

_____

What I ate today: _____

_____

_____

_____

_____

_____

_____

_____

_____

_____

_____

What did I do well? _____

_____

_____

_____

_____

_____

_____

_____

_____

_____

_____

Tomorrow I can eat more—smarter—5% more effectively by:

_____

_____

_____

_____

_____

_____

_____

_____

_____

_____

_____

Week 2—Day 5   Date:

		Ate:	Target:
Non-Starchy Vegetables	Ate: Target:	□□□□□□□□□□□	■■■■■■■■■■■
Seafood/Lean Meat/Egg Whites/Whey/Select Dairy	Ate: Target:	□□□□□□□□□□□	■■■■■
Flax Seeds/Nuts	Ate: Target:	□□□□□□□□□□□	■■■■■
Berries/Citrus Fruits	Ate: Target:	□□□□□□□□□□□	■■■■■
Legumes	Ate: Target:	□□□□□□□□□□□	
Other Fruits	Ate: Target:	□□□□□□□□□□□	
Most Dairy	Ate: Target:	□□□□□□□□□□□	
Fatty Meat/Oils	Ate: Target:	□□□□□□□□□□□	
Starchy Vegetables/Starch	Ate: Target:	□□□□□□□□□□□	
Sweets/Sweetened Drinks	Ate: Target:	□□□□□□□□□□□	

Today I am proud that I: _____

_____

_____

Today I noticed that eating more and exercising less—smarter—
had a positive impact on my life when: _____

_____

_____

_____

What I ate today: _____

_____

_____

_____

_____

_____

_____

_____

_____

_____

_____

What did I do well? _____

_____

_____

_____

_____

_____

_____

_____

_____

_____

_____

Tomorrow I can eat more—smarter—5% more effectively by:

_____

_____

_____

_____

_____

_____

_____

_____

_____

Week 2—Day 6   Date:

Non-Starchy Vegetables	Ate:	☐☐☐☐☐☐☐☐☐☐
	Target:	■■■■■■■■■■
Seafood/Lean Meat/Egg Whites/Whey/Select Dairy	Ate:	☐☐☐☐☐☐☐☐☐☐
	Target:	■■■■■
Flax Seeds/Nuts	Ate:	☐☐☐☐☐☐☐☐☐☐
	Target:	■■■■■
Berries/Citrus Fruits	Ate:	☐☐☐☐☐☐☐☐☐☐
	Target:	■■■■■
Legumes	Ate:	☐☐☐☐☐☐☐☐☐☐
	Target:	
Other Fruits	Ate:	☐☐☐☐☐☐☐☐☐☐
	Target:	
Most Dairy	Ate:	☐☐☐☐☐☐☐☐☐☐
	Target:	
Fatty Meat/Oils	Ate:	☐☐☐☐☐☐☐☐☐☐
	Target:	
Starchy Vegetables/Starch	Ate:	☐☐☐☐☐☐☐☐☐☐
	Target:	
Sweets/Sweetened Drinks	Ate:	☐☐☐☐☐☐☐☐☐☐
	Target:	

Today I am proud that I: _____

_____

_____

Today I noticed that eating more and exercising less—smarter—
had a positive impact on my life when: _____

_____

_____

_____

What I ate today: _____

_____

_____

_____

_____

_____

_____

_____

_____

What did I do well? _____

_____

_____

_____

_____

_____

_____

_____

_____

_____

Tomorrow I can eat more—smarter—5% more effectively by:

_____

_____

_____

_____

_____

_____

_____

_____

_____

Week 2—Day 7   Date:

Non-Starchy Vegetables	Ate:	☐☐☐☐☐☐☐☐☐☐☐
	Target:	■■■■■■■■■■
Seafood/Lean Meat/Egg Whites/Whey/Select Dairy	Ate:	☐☐☐☐☐☐☐☐☐☐☐
	Target:	■■■■■
Flax Seeds/Nuts	Ate:	☐☐☐☐☐☐☐☐☐☐☐
	Target:	■■■■■
Berries/Citrus Fruits	Ate:	☐☐☐☐☐☐☐☐☐☐☐
	Target:	■■■■■
Legumes	Ate:	☐☐☐☐☐☐☐☐☐☐☐
	Target:	
Other Fruits	Ate:	☐☐☐☐☐☐☐☐☐☐☐
	Target:	
Most Dairy	Ate:	☐☐☐☐☐☐☐☐☐☐☐
	Target:	
Fatty Meat/Oils	Ate:	☐☐☐☐☐☐☐☐☐☐☐
	Target:	
Starchy Vegetables/Starch	Ate:	☐☐☐☐☐☐☐☐☐☐☐
	Target:	
Sweets/Sweetened Drinks	Ate:	☐☐☐☐☐☐☐☐☐☐☐
	Target:	

Today I am proud that I: _____

_____

_____

Today I noticed that eating more and exercising less—smarter—
had a positive impact on my life when: _____

_____

_____

_____

What I ate today: _____
_____
_____
_____
_____
_____
_____
_____
_____
_____

What did I do well? _____
_____
_____
_____
_____
_____
_____
_____
_____
_____
_____

Tomorrow I can eat more—smarter—5% more effectively by:
_____
_____
_____
_____
_____
_____
_____
_____
_____
_____

Week 2 Eccentric Exercise   Date:

Home Option

		Add resistance?
Assisted Eccentric Squats	Resistance: _____	Y / N
Assisted Eccentric Pull-Ups	Resistance: _____	Y / N
Assisted Eccentric Push-Ups	Resistance: _____	Y / N
Assisted Eccentric Shoulder Press	Resistance: _____	Y / N

Gym Option

		Add resistance?
Eccentric Leg Presses	Resistance: _____	Y / N
Eccentric Rows	Resistance: _____	Y / N
Eccentric Check Presses	Resistance: _____	Y / N
Eccentric Shoulder Presses	Resistance: _____	Y / N

Week 1 Cardiovascular Exercise   Date:

		Add resistance?
10 Minutes of High-Quality Brief Cardiovascular Exercise	Resistance: _____	Y / N

Remember: It should be impossible to do more than six repetitions of each eccentric exercise per week. It should also be impossible to do more than six repetitions of brief cardiovascular exercise per week. If more repetitions are possible or more workouts are possible, then add resistance.

Notes: _____
_____
_____
_____
_____
_____
_____
_____
_____
_____

What did I do well? _____
_____
_____
_____
_____
_____
_____
_____
_____
_____

Next week I can exercise less—smarter—5% more effectively by:
_____
_____
_____
_____
_____
_____
_____
_____
_____

Week 3—Day 1   Date:

Non-Starchy Vegetables	Ate:	☐☐☐☐☐☐☐☐☐☐
	Target:	■■■■■■■■■■
Seafood/Lean Meat/Egg Whites/Whey/Select Dairy	Ate:	☐☐☐☐☐☐☐☐☐☐
	Target:	■■■■■
Flax Seeds/Nuts	Ate:	☐☐☐☐☐☐☐☐☐☐
	Target:	■■■■■
Berries/Citrus Fruits	Ate:	☐☐☐☐☐☐☐☐☐☐
	Target:	■■■■■
Legumes	Ate:	☐☐☐☐☐☐☐☐☐☐
	Target:	
Other Fruits	Ate:	☐☐☐☐☐☐☐☐☐☐
	Target:	
Most Dairy	Ate:	☐☐☐☐☐☐☐☐☐☐
	Target:	
Fatty Meat/Oils	Ate:	☐☐☐☐☐☐☐☐☐☐
	Target:	
Starchy Vegetables/Starch	Ate:	☐☐☐☐☐☐☐☐☐☐
	Target:	
Sweets/Sweetened Drinks	Ate:	☐☐☐☐☐☐☐☐☐☐
	Target:	

Today I am proud that I: _____

_____

_____

Today I noticed that eating more and exercising less—smarter—had a positive impact on my life when: _____

_____

_____

_____

What I ate today: _____

_____

_____

_____

_____

_____

_____

_____

_____

_____

What did I do well? _____

_____

_____

_____

_____

_____

_____

_____

_____

_____

_____

Tomorrow I can eat more—smarter—5% more effectively by:

_____

_____

_____

_____

_____

_____

_____

_____

_____

Week 3—Day 2   Date:

| Non-Starchy Vegetables | Ate: | ☐☐☐☐☐☐☐☐☐☐☐ |
| | Target: | ■■■■■■■■■■ |

| Seafood/Lean Meat/Egg Whites/Whey/Select Dairy | Ate: | ☐☐☐☐☐☐☐☐☐☐☐ |
| | Target: | ■■■■■ |

| Flax Seeds/Nuts | Ate: | ☐☐☐☐☐☐☐☐☐☐☐ |
| | Target: | ■■■■■ |

| Berries/Citrus Fruits | Ate: | ☐☐☐☐☐☐☐☐☐☐☐ |
| | Target: | ■■■■■ |

| Legumes | Ate: | ☐☐☐☐☐☐☐☐☐☐☐ |
| | Target: | |

| Other Fruits | Ate: | ☐☐☐☐☐☐☐☐☐☐☐ |
| | Target: | |

| Most Dairy | Ate: | ☐☐☐☐☐☐☐☐☐☐☐ |
| | Target: | |

| Fatty Meat/Oils | Ate: | ☐☐☐☐☐☐☐☐☐☐☐ |
| | Target: | |

| Starchy Vegetables/Starch | Ate: | ☐☐☐☐☐☐☐☐☐☐☐ |
| | Target: | |

| Sweets/Sweetened Drinks | Ate: | ☐☐☐☐☐☐☐☐☐☐☐ |
| | Target: | |

Today I am proud that I: _____

_____

_____

Today I noticed that eating more and exercising less—smarter—had a positive impact on my life when: _____

_____

_____

_____

What I ate today: _____

_____

_____

_____

_____

_____

_____

_____

_____

_____

_____

What did I do well? _____

_____

_____

_____

_____

_____

_____

_____

_____

_____

_____

Tomorrow I can eat more—smarter—5% more effectively by:

_____

_____

_____

_____

_____

_____

_____

_____

_____

Week 3—Day 3   Date:

Non-Starchy Vegetables	Ate:	☐☐☐☐☐☐☐☐☐☐☐
	Target:	■■■■■■■■■■
Seafood/Lean Meat/Egg Whites/Whey/Select Dairy	Ate:	☐☐☐☐☐☐☐☐☐☐☐
	Target:	■■■■■
Flax Seeds/Nuts	Ate:	☐☐☐☐☐☐☐☐☐☐☐
	Target:	■■■■■
Berries/Citrus Fruits	Ate:	☐☐☐☐☐☐☐☐☐☐☐
	Target:	■■■■■
Legumes	Ate:	☐☐☐☐☐☐☐☐☐☐☐
	Target:	
Other Fruits	Ate:	☐☐☐☐☐☐☐☐☐☐☐
	Target:	
Most Dairy	Ate:	☐☐☐☐☐☐☐☐☐☐☐
	Target:	
Fatty Meat/Oils	Ate:	☐☐☐☐☐☐☐☐☐☐☐
	Target:	
Starchy Vegetables/Starch	Ate:	☐☐☐☐☐☐☐☐☐☐☐
	Target:	
Sweets/Sweetened Drinks	Ate:	☐☐☐☐☐☐☐☐☐☐☐
	Target:	

Today I am proud that I: _____

_____

_____

Today I noticed that eating more and exercising less—smarter—
had a positive impact on my life when: _____

_____

_____

_____

What I ate today: _____

_____

_____

_____

_____

_____

_____

_____

_____

_____

What did I do well? _____

_____

_____

_____

_____

_____

_____

_____

_____

_____

Tomorrow I can eat more—smarter—5% more effectively by:

_____

_____

_____

_____

_____

_____

_____

_____

_____

Week 3—Day 4   Date:

		Counts
Non-Starchy Vegetables	Ate:	☐☐☐☐☐☐☐☐☐☐☐
	Target:	■■■■■■■■■■■
Seafood/Lean Meat/Egg Whites/Whey/Select Dairy	Ate:	☐☐☐☐☐☐☐☐☐☐☐
	Target:	■■■■■■
Flax Seeds/Nuts	Ate:	☐☐☐☐☐☐☐☐☐☐☐
	Target:	■■■■■■
Berries/Citrus Fruits	Ate:	☐☐☐☐☐☐☐☐☐☐☐
	Target:	■■■■■■
Legumes	Ate:	☐☐☐☐☐☐☐☐☐☐☐
	Target:	
Other Fruits	Ate:	☐☐☐☐☐☐☐☐☐☐☐
	Target:	
Most Dairy	Ate:	☐☐☐☐☐☐☐☐☐☐☐
	Target:	
Fatty Meat/Oils	Ate:	☐☐☐☐☐☐☐☐☐☐☐
	Target:	
Starchy Vegetables/Starch	Ate:	☐☐☐☐☐☐☐☐☐☐☐
	Target:	
Sweets/Sweetened Drinks	Ate:	☐☐☐☐☐☐☐☐☐☐☐
	Target:	

Today I am proud that I: _____
_____
_____

Today I noticed that eating more and exercising less—smarter—
had a positive impact on my life when: _____
_____
_____
_____

What I ate today: _____

_____

_____

_____

_____

_____

_____

_____

_____

_____

What did I do well? _____

_____

_____

_____

_____

_____

_____

_____

_____

_____

Tomorrow I can eat more—smarter—5% more effectively by:

_____

_____

_____

_____

_____

_____

_____

_____

Week 3—Day 5   Date:

Non-Starchy Vegetables	Ate:	☐☐☐☐☐☐☐☐☐☐
	Target:	■■■■■■■■■■
Seafood/Lean Meat/Egg Whites/Whey/Select Dairy	Ate:	☐☐☐☐☐☐☐☐☐☐
	Target:	■■■■■
Flax Seeds/Nuts	Ate:	☐☐☐☐☐☐☐☐☐☐
	Target:	■■■■■
Berries/Citrus Fruits	Ate:	☐☐☐☐☐☐☐☐☐☐
	Target:	■■■■■
Legumes	Ate:	☐☐☐☐☐☐☐☐☐☐
	Target:	
Other Fruits	Ate:	☐☐☐☐☐☐☐☐☐☐
	Target:	
Most Dairy	Ate:	☐☐☐☐☐☐☐☐☐☐
	Target:	
Fatty Meat/Oils	Ate:	☐☐☐☐☐☐☐☐☐☐
	Target:	
Starchy Vegetables/Starch	Ate:	☐☐☐☐☐☐☐☐☐☐
	Target:	
Sweets/Sweetened Drinks	Ate:	☐☐☐☐☐☐☐☐☐☐
	Target:	

Today I am proud that I: _____
_____
_____

Today I noticed that eating more and exercising less—smarter—
had a positive impact on my life when: _____
_____
_____
_____

What I ate today: _____

_____

_____

_____

_____

_____

_____

_____

_____

_____

What did I do well? _____

_____

_____

_____

_____

_____

_____

_____

_____

_____

_____

Tomorrow I can eat more—smarter—5% more effectively by:

_____

_____

_____

_____

_____

_____

_____

_____

_____

_____

Week 3—Day 6   Date:

Non-Starchy Vegetables	Ate:	☐☐☐☐☐☐☐☐☐☐☐
	Target:	■■■■■■■■■■■
Seafood/Lean Meat/Egg Whites/Whey/Select Dairy	Ate:	☐☐☐☐☐☐☐☐☐☐☐
	Target:	■■■■■
Flax Seeds/Nuts	Ate:	☐☐☐☐☐☐☐☐☐☐☐
	Target:	■■■■■
Berries/Citrus Fruits	Ate:	☐☐☐☐☐☐☐☐☐☐☐
	Target:	■■■■■
Legumes	Ate:	☐☐☐☐☐☐☐☐☐☐☐
	Target:	
Other Fruits	Ate:	☐☐☐☐☐☐☐☐☐☐☐
	Target:	
Most Dairy	Ate:	☐☐☐☐☐☐☐☐☐☐☐
	Target:	
Fatty Meat/Oils	Ate:	☐☐☐☐☐☐☐☐☐☐☐
	Target:	
Starchy Vegetables/Starch	Ate:	☐☐☐☐☐☐☐☐☐☐☐
	Target:	
Sweets/Sweetened Drinks	Ate:	☐☐☐☐☐☐☐☐☐☐☐
	Target:	

Today I am proud that I: _____

_____

_____

Today I noticed that eating more and exercising less—smarter—had a positive impact on my life when: _____

_____

_____

_____

What I ate today: _____

_____

_____

_____

_____

_____

_____

_____

_____

_____

What did I do well? _____

_____

_____

_____

_____

_____

_____

_____

_____

_____

_____

Tomorrow I can eat more—smarter—5% more effectively by:

_____

_____

_____

_____

_____

_____

_____

_____

_____

Week 3—Day 7   Date:

Non-Starchy Vegetables	Ate:	☐☐☐☐☐☐☐☐☐☐
	Target:	■■■■■■■■■■
Seafood/Lean Meat/Egg Whites/Whey/Select Dairy	Ate:	☐☐☐☐☐☐☐☐☐☐
	Target:	■■■■■
Flax Seeds/Nuts	Ate:	☐☐☐☐☐☐☐☐☐☐
	Target:	■■■■■
Berries/Citrus Fruits	Ate:	☐☐☐☐☐☐☐☐☐☐
	Target:	■■■■■
Legumes	Ate:	☐☐☐☐☐☐☐☐☐☐
	Target:	
Other Fruits	Ate:	☐☐☐☐☐☐☐☐☐☐
	Target:	
Most Dairy	Ate:	☐☐☐☐☐☐☐☐☐☐
	Target:	
Fatty Meat/Oils	Ate:	☐☐☐☐☐☐☐☐☐☐
	Target:	
Starchy Vegetables/Starch	Ate:	☐☐☐☐☐☐☐☐☐☐
	Target:	
Sweets/Sweetened Drinks	Ate:	☐☐☐☐☐☐☐☐☐☐
	Target:	

Today I am proud that I: _____

_____

_____

Today I noticed that eating more and exercising less—smarter—
had a positive impact on my life when: _____

_____

_____

_____

What I ate today: _____

_____

_____

_____

_____

_____

_____

_____

_____

_____

What did I do well? _____

_____

_____

_____

_____

_____

_____

_____

_____

_____

Tomorrow I can eat more—smarter—5% more effectively by:

_____

_____

_____

_____

_____

_____

_____

_____

_____

Week 3 Eccentric Exercise   Date:

Home Option

		Add resistance?
Assisted Eccentric Squats	Resistance: _____	Y / N
Assisted Eccentric Pull-Ups	Resistance: _____	Y / N
Assisted Eccentric Push-Ups	Resistance: _____	Y / N
Assisted Eccentric Shoulder Press	Resistance: _____	Y / N

Gym Option

		Add resistance?
Eccentric Leg Presses	Resistance: _____	Y / N
Eccentric Rows	Resistance: _____	Y / N
Eccentric Check Presses	Resistance: _____	Y / N
Eccentric Shoulder Presses	Resistance: _____	Y / N

Week 1 Cardiovascular Exercise   Date:

		Add resistance?
10 Minutes of High-Quality Brief Cardiovascular Exercise	Resistance: _____	Y / N

Remember: It should be impossible to do more than six repetitions of each eccentric exercise per week. It should also be impossible to do more than six repetitions of brief cardiovascular exercise per week. If more repetitions are possible or more workouts are possible, then add resistance.

Notes: _____
_____
_____
_____
_____
_____
_____
_____
_____
_____
_____

What did I do well? _____
_____
_____
_____
_____
_____
_____
_____
_____
_____
_____

Next week I can exercise less—smarter—5% more effectively by:
_____
_____
_____
_____
_____
_____
_____
_____
_____

Week 4—Day 1   Date:

Non-Starchy Vegetables	Ate:	☐☐☐☐☐☐☐☐☐☐☐
	Target:	■■■■■■■■■■
Seafood/Lean Meat/Egg Whites/Whey/Select Dairy	Ate:	☐☐☐☐☐☐☐☐☐☐☐
	Target:	■■■■■
Flax Seeds/Nuts	Ate:	☐☐☐☐☐☐☐☐☐☐☐
	Target:	■■■■■
Berries/Citrus Fruits	Ate:	☐☐☐☐☐☐☐☐☐☐☐
	Target:	■■■■■
Legumes	Ate:	☐☐☐☐☐☐☐☐☐☐☐
	Target:	
Other Fruits	Ate:	☐☐☐☐☐☐☐☐☐☐☐
	Target:	
Most Dairy	Ate:	☐☐☐☐☐☐☐☐☐☐☐
	Target:	
Fatty Meat/Oils	Ate:	☐☐☐☐☐☐☐☐☐☐☐
	Target:	
Starchy Vegetables/Starch	Ate:	☐☐☐☐☐☐☐☐☐☐☐
	Target:	
Sweets/Sweetened Drinks	Ate:	☐☐☐☐☐☐☐☐☐☐☐
	Target:	

Today I am proud that I: _____

_____

_____

Today I noticed that eating more and exercising less—smarter—
had a positive impact on my life when: _____

_____

_____

_____

What I ate today: _____

_____

_____

_____

_____

_____

_____

_____

_____

_____

What did I do well? _____

_____

_____

_____

_____

_____

_____

_____

_____

_____

Tomorrow I can eat more—smarter—5% more effectively by:

_____

_____

_____

_____

_____

_____

_____

_____

_____

Week 4—Day 2   Date:

Non-Starchy Vegetables — Ate: ☐☐☐☐☐☐☐☐☐☐☐ Target: ■■■■■■■■■■

Seafood/Lean Meat/Egg Whites/Whey/Select Dairy — Ate: ☐☐☐☐☐☐☐☐☐☐☐ Target: ■■■■■■

Flax Seeds/Nuts — Ate: ☐☐☐☐☐☐☐☐☐☐☐ Target: ■■■■■■

Berries/Citrus Fruits — Ate: ☐☐☐☐☐☐☐☐☐☐☐ Target: ■■■■■■

Legumes — Ate: ☐☐☐☐☐☐☐☐☐☐☐ Target:

Other Fruits — Ate: ☐☐☐☐☐☐☐☐☐☐☐ Target:

Most Dairy — Ate: ☐☐☐☐☐☐☐☐☐☐☐ Target:

Fatty Meat/Oils — Ate: ☐☐☐☐☐☐☐☐☐☐☐ Target:

Starchy Vegetables/Starch — Ate: ☐☐☐☐☐☐☐☐☐☐☐ Target:

Sweets/Sweetened Drinks — Ate: ☐☐☐☐☐☐☐☐☐☐☐ Target:

Today I am proud that I: _____

_____

_____

Today I noticed that eating more and exercising less—smarter—had a positive impact on my life when: _____

_____

_____

_____

What I ate today: _____

_____

_____

_____

_____

_____

_____

_____

_____

_____

What did I do well? _____

_____

_____

_____

_____

_____

_____

_____

_____

_____

Tomorrow I can eat more—smarter—5% more effectively by:

_____

_____

_____

_____

_____

_____

_____

_____

_____

Week 4—Day 3   Date:

Non-Starchy Vegetables	Ate:	☐☐☐☐☐☐☐☐☐☐☐
	Target:	■■■■■■■■■■
Seafood/Lean Meat/Egg Whites/Whey/Select Dairy	Ate:	☐☐☐☐☐☐☐☐☐☐☐
	Target:	■■■■■
Flax Seeds/Nuts	Ate:	☐☐☐☐☐☐☐☐☐☐☐
	Target:	■■■■■
Berries/Citrus Fruits	Ate:	☐☐☐☐☐☐☐☐☐☐☐
	Target:	■■■■■
Legumes	Ate:	☐☐☐☐☐☐☐☐☐☐☐
	Target:	
Other Fruits	Ate:	☐☐☐☐☐☐☐☐☐☐☐
	Target:	
Most Dairy	Ate:	☐☐☐☐☐☐☐☐☐☐☐
	Target:	
Fatty Meat/Oils	Ate:	☐☐☐☐☐☐☐☐☐☐☐
	Target:	
Starchy Vegetables/Starch	Ate:	☐☐☐☐☐☐☐☐☐☐☐
	Target:	
Sweets/Sweetened Drinks	Ate:	☐☐☐☐☐☐☐☐☐☐☐
	Target:	

Today I am proud that I: _____

_____

_____

Today I noticed that eating more and exercising less—smarter—
had a positive impact on my life when: _____

_____

_____

_____

What I ate today: _____
_____
_____
_____
_____
_____
_____
_____
_____
_____
_____

What did I do well? _____
_____
_____
_____
_____
_____
_____
_____
_____
_____
_____

Tomorrow I can eat more—smarter—5% more effectively by:
_____
_____
_____
_____
_____
_____
_____
_____
_____

Week 4—Day 4   Date:

Non-Starchy Vegetables	Ate:	☐☐☐☐☐☐☐☐☐☐☐
	Target:	■■■■■■■■■■
Seafood/Lean Meat/Egg Whites/Whey/Select Dairy	Ate:	☐☐☐☐☐☐☐☐☐☐☐
	Target:	■■■■■
Flax Seeds/Nuts	Ate:	☐☐☐☐☐☐☐☐☐☐☐
	Target:	■■■■■
Berries/Citrus Fruits	Ate:	☐☐☐☐☐☐☐☐☐☐☐
	Target:	■■■■■
Legumes	Ate:	☐☐☐☐☐☐☐☐☐☐☐
	Target:	
Other Fruits	Ate:	☐☐☐☐☐☐☐☐☐☐☐
	Target:	
Most Dairy	Ate:	☐☐☐☐☐☐☐☐☐☐☐
	Target:	
Fatty Meat/Oils	Ate:	☐☐☐☐☐☐☐☐☐☐☐
	Target:	
Starchy Vegetables/Starch	Ate:	☐☐☐☐☐☐☐☐☐☐☐
	Target:	
Sweets/Sweetened Drinks	Ate:	☐☐☐☐☐☐☐☐☐☐☐
	Target:	

Today I am proud that I: _____

_____

_____

Today I noticed that eating more and exercising less—smarter—
had a positive impact on my life when: _____

_____

_____

_____

What I ate today: _____

_____

_____

_____

_____

_____

_____

_____

_____

_____

What did I do well? _____

_____

_____

_____

_____

_____

_____

_____

_____

_____

Tomorrow I can eat more—smarter—5% more effectively by:

_____

_____

_____

_____

_____

_____

_____

_____

_____

Week 4—Day 5   Date:

Non-Starchy Vegetables	Ate:	☐☐☐☐☐☐☐☐☐☐☐☐
	Target:	■■■■■■■■■■
Seafood/Lean Meat/Egg Whites/Whey/Select Dairy	Ate:	☐☐☐☐☐☐☐☐☐☐☐☐
	Target:	■■■■■
Flax Seeds/Nuts	Ate:	☐☐☐☐☐☐☐☐☐☐☐☐
	Target:	■■■■■
Berries/Citrus Fruits	Ate:	☐☐☐☐☐☐☐☐☐☐☐☐
	Target:	■■■■■
Legumes	Ate:	☐☐☐☐☐☐☐☐☐☐☐
	Target:	
Other Fruits	Ate:	☐☐☐☐☐☐☐☐☐☐☐
	Target:	
Most Dairy	Ate:	☐☐☐☐☐☐☐☐☐☐☐
	Target:	
Fatty Meat/Oils	Ate:	☐☐☐☐☐☐☐☐☐☐☐
	Target:	
Starchy Vegetables/Starch	Ate:	☐☐☐☐☐☐☐☐☐☐☐
	Target:	
Sweets/Sweetened Drinks	Ate:	☐☐☐☐☐☐☐☐☐☐☐
	Target:	

Today I am proud that I: _____

_____

_____

Today I noticed that eating more and exercising less—smarter—
had a positive impact on my life when: _____

_____

_____

_____

What I ate today: _____

_____

_____

_____

_____

_____

_____

_____

_____

_____

What did I do well? _____

_____

_____

_____

_____

_____

_____

_____

_____

_____

Tomorrow I can eat more—smarter—5% more effectively by:

_____

_____

_____

_____

_____

_____

_____

_____

_____

Week 4—Day 6   Date:

Non-Starchy Vegetables	Ate:	☐☐☐☐☐☐☐☐☐☐
	Target:	■■■■■■■■■
Seafood/Lean Meat/Egg Whites/Whey/Select Dairy	Ate:	☐☐☐☐☐☐☐☐☐☐
	Target:	■■■■■
Flax Seeds/Nuts	Ate:	☐☐☐☐☐☐☐☐☐☐
	Target:	■■■■■
Berries/Citrus Fruits	Ate:	☐☐☐☐☐☐☐☐☐☐
	Target:	■■■■■
Legumes	Ate:	☐☐☐☐☐☐☐☐☐☐
	Target:	
Other Fruits	Ate:	☐☐☐☐☐☐☐☐☐☐
	Target:	
Most Dairy	Ate:	☐☐☐☐☐☐☐☐☐☐
	Target:	
Fatty Meat/Oils	Ate:	☐☐☐☐☐☐☐☐☐☐
	Target:	
Starchy Vegetables/Starch	Ate:	☐☐☐☐☐☐☐☐☐☐
	Target:	
Sweets/Sweetened Drinks	Ate:	☐☐☐☐☐☐☐☐☐☐
	Target:	

Today I am proud that I: _____

_____

_____

Today I noticed that eating more and exercising less—smarter—
had a positive impact on my life when: _____

_____

_____

_____

What I ate today: _____
_____
_____
_____
_____
_____
_____
_____
_____
_____
_____

What did I do well? _____
_____
_____
_____
_____
_____
_____
_____
_____
_____
_____

Tomorrow I can eat more—smarter—5% more effectively by:
_____
_____
_____
_____
_____
_____
_____
_____
_____

Week 4—Day 7   Date:

Non-Starchy Vegetables	Ate:	☐☐☐☐☐☐☐☐☐☐☐☐
	Target:	■■■■■■■■■■
Seafood/Lean Meat/Egg Whites/Whey/Select Dairy	Ate:	☐☐☐☐☐☐☐☐☐☐☐☐
	Target:	■■■■■
Flax Seeds/Nuts	Ate:	☐☐☐☐☐☐☐☐☐☐☐☐
	Target:	■■■■■
Berries/Citrus Fruits	Ate:	☐☐☐☐☐☐☐☐☐☐☐☐
	Target:	■■■■■
Legumes	Ate:	☐☐☐☐☐☐☐☐☐☐☐
	Target:	
Other Fruits	Ate:	☐☐☐☐☐☐☐☐☐☐☐
	Target:	
Most Dairy	Ate:	☐☐☐☐☐☐☐☐☐☐☐
	Target:	
Fatty Meat/Oils	Ate:	☐☐☐☐☐☐☐☐☐☐☐
	Target:	
Starchy Vegetables/Starch	Ate:	☐☐☐☐☐☐☐☐☐☐☐
	Target:	
Sweets/Sweetened Drinks	Ate:	☐☐☐☐☐☐☐☐☐☐☐
	Target:	

Today I am proud that I: _____

_____

_____

Today I noticed that eating more and exercising less—smarter—
had a positive impact on my life when: _____

_____

_____

_____

What I ate today: _____
_____
_____
_____
_____
_____
_____
_____
_____
_____

What did I do well? _____
_____
_____
_____
_____
_____
_____
_____
_____
_____

Tomorrow I can eat more—smarter—5% more effectively by:
_____
_____
_____
_____
_____
_____
_____
_____
_____

Week 4 Eccentric Exercise   Date:

Home Option

			Add resistance?
Assisted Eccentric Squats	Resistance:	_____	Y / N
Assisted Eccentric Pull-Ups	Resistance:	_____	Y / N
Assisted Eccentric Push-Ups	Resistance:	_____	Y / N
Assisted Eccentric Shoulder Press	Resistance:	_____	Y / N

Gym Option

			Add resistance?
Eccentric Leg Presses	Resistance:	_____	Y / N
Eccentric Rows	Resistance:	_____	Y / N
Eccentric Check Presses	Resistance:	_____	Y / N
Eccentric Shoulder Presses	Resistance:	_____	Y / N

Week 1 Cardiovascular Exercise   Date:

			Add resistance?
10 Minutes of High-Quality Brief Cardiovascular Exercise	Resistance:	_____	Y / N

Remember: It should be impossible to do more than six repetitions of each eccentric exercise per week. It should also be impossible to do more than six repetitions of brief cardiovascular exercise per week. If more repetitions are possible or more workouts are possible, then add resistance.

Notes: _____
_____
_____
_____
_____
_____
_____
_____
_____
_____
_____
_____

What did I do well? _____
_____
_____
_____
_____
_____
_____
_____
_____
_____
_____
_____

Next week I can exercise less—smarter—5% more effectively by:
_____
_____
_____
_____
_____
_____
_____
_____
_____
_____
_____

Week 5—Day 1   Date:

Non-Starchy Vegetables	Ate:	☐☐☐☐☐☐☐☐☐☐☐
	Target:	■■■■■■■■■
Seafood/Lean Meat/Egg Whites/Whey/Select Dairy	Ate:	☐☐☐☐☐☐☐☐☐☐☐
	Target:	■■■■■
Flax Seeds/Nuts	Ate:	☐☐☐☐☐☐☐☐☐☐☐
	Target:	■■■■■
Berries/Citrus Fruits	Ate:	☐☐☐☐☐☐☐☐☐☐☐
	Target:	■■■■■
Legumes	Ate:	☐☐☐☐☐☐☐☐☐☐☐
	Target:	
Other Fruits	Ate:	☐☐☐☐☐☐☐☐☐☐☐
	Target:	
Most Dairy	Ate:	☐☐☐☐☐☐☐☐☐☐☐
	Target:	
Fatty Meat/Oils	Ate:	☐☐☐☐☐☐☐☐☐☐☐
	Target:	
Starchy Vegetables/Starch	Ate:	☐☐☐☐☐☐☐☐☐☐☐
	Target:	
Sweets/Sweetened Drinks	Ate:	☐☐☐☐☐☐☐☐☐☐☐
	Target:	

Today I am proud that I: _____

_____

_____

Today I noticed that eating more and exercising less—smarter—
had a positive impact on my life when: _____

_____

_____

_____

What I ate today: _____
_____
_____
_____
_____
_____
_____
_____
_____
_____

What did I do well? _____
_____
_____
_____
_____
_____
_____
_____
_____
_____

Tomorrow I can eat more—smarter—5% more effectively by:
_____
_____
_____
_____
_____
_____
_____
_____
_____

Week 5—Day 2   Date:

Non-Starchy Vegetables	Ate:	☐☐☐☐☐☐☐☐☐☐☐
	Target:	■■■■■■■■■■
Seafood/Lean Meat/Egg Whites/Whey/Select Dairy	Ate:	☐☐☐☐☐☐☐☐☐☐☐
	Target:	■■■■■
Flax Seeds/Nuts	Ate:	☐☐☐☐☐☐☐☐☐☐☐
	Target:	■■■■■
Berries/Citrus Fruits	Ate:	☐☐☐☐☐☐☐☐☐☐☐
	Target:	■■■■■
Legumes	Ate:	☐☐☐☐☐☐☐☐☐☐☐
	Target:	
Other Fruits	Ate:	☐☐☐☐☐☐☐☐☐☐☐
	Target:	
Most Dairy	Ate:	☐☐☐☐☐☐☐☐☐☐☐
	Target:	
Fatty Meat/Oils	Ate:	☐☐☐☐☐☐☐☐☐☐☐
	Target:	
Starchy Vegetables/Starch	Ate:	☐☐☐☐☐☐☐☐☐☐☐
	Target:	
Sweets/Sweetened Drinks	Ate:	☐☐☐☐☐☐☐☐☐☐☐
	Target:	

Today I am proud that I: _____

_____

_____

Today I noticed that eating more and exercising less—smarter—
had a positive impact on my life when: _____

_____

_____

_____

What I ate today: _____

_____

_____

_____

_____

_____

_____

_____

_____

What did I do well? _____

_____

_____

_____

_____

_____

_____

_____

_____

_____

Tomorrow I can eat more—smarter—5% more effectively by:

_____

_____

_____

_____

_____

_____

_____

_____

_____

Week 5—Day 3   Date:

Non-Starchy Vegetables	Ate:	☐☐☐☐☐☐☐☐☐☐
	Target:	■■■■■■■■■■
Seafood/Lean Meat/Egg Whites/Whey/Select Dairy	Ate:	☐☐☐☐☐☐☐☐☐☐
	Target:	■■■■■
Flax Seeds/Nuts	Ate:	☐☐☐☐☐☐☐☐☐☐
	Target:	■■■■■
Berries/Citrus Fruits	Ate:	☐☐☐☐☐☐☐☐☐☐
	Target:	■■■■■
Legumes	Ate:	☐☐☐☐☐☐☐☐☐☐
	Target:	
Other Fruits	Ate:	☐☐☐☐☐☐☐☐☐☐
	Target:	
Most Dairy	Ate:	☐☐☐☐☐☐☐☐☐☐
	Target:	
Fatty Meat/Oils	Ate:	☐☐☐☐☐☐☐☐☐☐
	Target:	
Starchy Vegetables/Starch	Ate:	☐☐☐☐☐☐☐☐☐☐
	Target:	
Sweets/Sweetened Drinks	Ate:	☐☐☐☐☐☐☐☐☐☐
	Target:	

Today I am proud that I: _____

_____

_____

Today I noticed that eating more and exercising less—smarter—had a positive impact on my life when: _____

_____

_____

_____

What I ate today: _____

_____

_____

_____

_____

_____

_____

_____

_____

_____

What did I do well? _____

_____

_____

_____

_____

_____

_____

_____

_____

_____

Tomorrow I can eat more—smarter—5% more effectively by:

_____

_____

_____

_____

_____

_____

_____

_____

_____

Week 5—Day 4   Date:

		Ate:	☐☐☐☐☐☐☐☐☐☐
Non-Starchy Vegetables		Target:	■■■■■■■■■■
Seafood/Lean Meat/Egg Whites/Whey/Select Dairy		Ate:	☐☐☐☐☐☐☐☐☐☐
		Target:	■■■■■■
Flax Seeds/Nuts		Ate:	☐☐☐☐☐☐☐☐☐☐
		Target:	■■■■■■
Berries/Citrus Fruits		Ate:	☐☐☐☐☐☐☐☐☐☐
		Target:	■■■■■■
Legumes		Ate:	☐☐☐☐☐☐☐☐☐☐
		Target:	
Other Fruits		Ate:	☐☐☐☐☐☐☐☐☐☐
		Target:	
Most Dairy		Ate:	☐☐☐☐☐☐☐☐☐☐
		Target:	
Fatty Meat/Oils		Ate:	☐☐☐☐☐☐☐☐☐☐
		Target:	
Starchy Vegetables/Starch		Ate:	☐☐☐☐☐☐☐☐☐☐
		Target:	
Sweets/Sweetened Drinks		Ate:	☐☐☐☐☐☐☐☐☐☐
		Target:	

Today I am proud that I: _____

_____

_____

Today I noticed that eating more and exercising less—smarter—had a positive impact on my life when: _____

_____

_____

_____

What I ate today: _____
_____
_____
_____
_____
_____
_____
_____
_____
_____

What did I do well? _____
_____
_____
_____
_____
_____
_____
_____
_____
_____

Tomorrow I can eat more—smarter—5% more effectively by:
_____
_____
_____
_____
_____
_____
_____
_____
_____

Week 5—Day 5   Date:

Non-Starchy Vegetables	Ate:	☐☐☐☐☐☐☐☐☐☐
	Target:	■■■■■■■■■■
Seafood/Lean Meat/Egg Whites/Whey/Select Dairy	Ate:	☐☐☐☐☐☐☐☐☐☐
	Target:	■■■■■
Flax Seeds/Nuts	Ate:	☐☐☐☐☐☐☐☐☐☐
	Target:	■■■■■
Berries/Citrus Fruits	Ate:	☐☐☐☐☐☐☐☐☐☐
	Target:	■■■■■
Legumes	Ate:	☐☐☐☐☐☐☐☐☐☐
	Target:	
Other Fruits	Ate:	☐☐☐☐☐☐☐☐☐☐
	Target:	
Most Dairy	Ate:	☐☐☐☐☐☐☐☐☐☐
	Target:	
Fatty Meat/Oils	Ate:	☐☐☐☐☐☐☐☐☐☐
	Target:	
Starchy Vegetables/Starch	Ate:	☐☐☐☐☐☐☐☐☐☐
	Target:	
Sweets/Sweetened Drinks	Ate:	☐☐☐☐☐☐☐☐☐☐
	Target:	

Today I am proud that I: _____

_____

_____

Today I noticed that eating more and exercising less—smarter—
had a positive impact on my life when: _____

_____

_____

_____

What I ate today: _____

_____

_____

_____

_____

_____

_____

_____

_____

_____

What did I do well? _____

_____

_____

_____

_____

_____

_____

_____

_____

_____

_____

Tomorrow I can eat more—smarter—5% more effectively by:

_____

_____

_____

_____

_____

_____

_____

_____

_____

_____

Week 5—Day 6   Date:

Non-Starchy Vegetables	Ate:	☐☐☐☐☐☐☐☐☐☐☐
	Target:	■■■■■■■■■■
Seafood/Lean Meat/Egg Whites/Whey/Select Dairy	Ate:	☐☐☐☐☐☐☐☐☐☐☐
	Target:	■■■■■■
Flax Seeds/Nuts	Ate:	☐☐☐☐☐☐☐☐☐☐☐
	Target:	■■■■■■
Berries/Citrus Fruits	Ate:	☐☐☐☐☐☐☐☐☐☐☐
	Target:	■■■■■■
Legumes	Ate:	☐☐☐☐☐☐☐☐☐☐☐
	Target:	
Other Fruits	Ate:	☐☐☐☐☐☐☐☐☐☐☐
	Target:	
Most Dairy	Ate:	☐☐☐☐☐☐☐☐☐☐☐
	Target:	
Fatty Meat/Oils	Ate:	☐☐☐☐☐☐☐☐☐☐☐
	Target:	
Starchy Vegetables/Starch	Ate:	☐☐☐☐☐☐☐☐☐☐☐
	Target:	
Sweets/Sweetened Drinks	Ate:	☐☐☐☐☐☐☐☐☐☐☐
	Target:	

Today I am proud that I: _____

_____

_____

Today I noticed that eating more and exercising less—smarter—had a positive impact on my life when: _____

_____

_____

_____

What I ate today: _____

_____

_____

_____

_____

_____

_____

_____

_____

_____

What did I do well? _____

_____

_____

_____

_____

_____

_____

_____

_____

_____

Tomorrow I can eat more—smarter—5% more effectively by:

_____

_____

_____

_____

_____

_____

_____

_____

_____

Week 5—Day 7   Date:

Non-Starchy Vegetables
Ate: ☐☐☐☐☐☐☐☐☐☐☐☐
Target: ■■■■■■■■■■■■

Seafood/Lean Meat/Egg Whites/Whey/Select Dairy
Ate: ☐☐☐☐☐☐☐☐☐☐☐☐
Target: ■■■■■■

Flax Seeds/Nuts
Ate: ☐☐☐☐☐☐☐☐☐☐☐☐
Target: ■■■■■■

Berries/Citrus Fruits
Ate: ☐☐☐☐☐☐☐☐☐☐☐☐
Target: ■■■■■■

Legumes
Ate: ☐☐☐☐☐☐☐☐☐☐☐☐
Target:

Other Fruits
Ate: ☐☐☐☐☐☐☐☐☐☐☐☐
Target:

Most Dairy
Ate: ☐☐☐☐☐☐☐☐☐☐☐☐
Target:

Fatty Meat/Oils
Ate: ☐☐☐☐☐☐☐☐☐☐☐☐
Target:

Starchy Vegetables/Starch
Ate: ☐☐☐☐☐☐☐☐☐☐☐☐
Target:

Sweets/Sweetened Drinks
Ate: ☐☐☐☐☐☐☐☐☐☐☐☐
Target:

Today I am proud that I: _____
_____
_____

Today I noticed that eating more and exercising less—smarter—had a positive impact on my life when: _____
_____
_____
_____

What I ate today: _____

_____

_____

_____

_____

_____

_____

_____

_____

_____

_____

What did I do well? _____

_____

_____

_____

_____

_____

_____

_____

_____

_____

_____

Tomorrow I can eat more—smarter—5% more effectively by:

_____

_____

_____

_____

_____

_____

_____

_____

_____

_____

Week 5 Eccentric Exercise   Date:

Home Option

		Add resistance?
Assisted Eccentric Squats	Resistance: _____	Y / N
Assisted Eccentric Pull-Ups	Resistance: _____	Y / N
Assisted Eccentric Push-Ups	Resistance: _____	Y / N
Assisted Eccentric Shoulder Press	Resistance: _____	Y / N

Gym Option

		Add resistance?
Eccentric Leg Presses	Resistance: _____	Y / N
Eccentric Rows	Resistance: _____	Y / N
Eccentric Check Presses	Resistance: _____	Y / N
Eccentric Shoulder Presses	Resistance: _____	Y / N

Week 1 Cardiovascular Exercise   Date:

		Add resistance?
10 Minutes of High-Quality Brief Cardiovascular Exercise	Resistance: _____	Y / N

Remember: It should be impossible to do more than six repetitions of each eccentric exercise per week. It should also be impossible to do more than six repetitions of brief cardiovascular exercise per week. If more repetitions are possible or more workouts are possible, then add resistance.

Notes: _____
_____
_____
_____
_____
_____
_____
_____
_____
_____
_____

What did I do well? _____
_____
_____
_____
_____
_____
_____
_____
_____
_____
_____

Next week I can exercise less—smarter—5% more effectively by:
_____
_____
_____
_____
_____
_____
_____
_____
_____
_____

Week 6—Day 1   Date:

Non-Starchy Vegetables	Ate:	☐☐☐☐☐☐☐☐☐☐☐☐
	Target:	■■■■■■■■■■■■
Seafood/Lean Meat/Egg Whites/Whey/Select Dairy	Ate:	☐☐☐☐☐☐☐☐☐☐☐☐
	Target:	■■■■■■
Flax Seeds/Nuts	Ate:	☐☐☐☐☐☐☐☐☐☐☐☐
	Target:	■■■■■
Berries/Citrus Fruits	Ate:	☐☐☐☐☐☐☐☐☐☐☐☐
	Target:	■■■■■
Legumes	Ate:	☐☐☐☐☐☐☐☐☐☐☐
	Target:	
Other Fruits	Ate:	☐☐☐☐☐☐☐☐☐☐☐
	Target:	
Most Dairy	Ate:	☐☐☐☐☐☐☐☐☐☐☐
	Target:	
Fatty Meat/Oils	Ate:	☐☐☐☐☐☐☐☐☐☐☐
	Target:	
Starchy Vegetables/Starch	Ate:	☐☐☐☐☐☐☐☐☐☐☐
	Target:	
Sweets/Sweetened Drinks	Ate:	☐☐☐☐☐☐☐☐☐☐☐
	Target:	

Today I am proud that I: _____

_____

_____

Today I noticed that eating more and exercising less—smarter—
had a positive impact on my life when: _____

_____

_____

_____

What I ate today: _____
_____
_____
_____
_____
_____
_____
_____
_____
_____
_____

What did I do well? _____
_____
_____
_____
_____
_____
_____
_____
_____
_____
_____

Tomorrow I can eat more—smarter—5% more effectively by:
_____
_____
_____
_____
_____
_____
_____
_____
_____
_____

Week 6—Day 2   Date:

Non-Starchy Vegetables	Ate:	☐☐☐☐☐☐☐☐☐☐
	Target:	■■■■■■■■■■
Seafood/Lean Meat/Egg Whites/Whey/Select Dairy	Ate:	☐☐☐☐☐☐☐☐☐☐
	Target:	■■■■■■
Flax Seeds/Nuts	Ate:	☐☐☐☐☐☐☐☐☐☐
	Target:	■■■■■■
Berries/Citrus Fruits	Ate:	☐☐☐☐☐☐☐☐☐☐
	Target:	■■■■■■
Legumes	Ate:	☐☐☐☐☐☐☐☐☐☐
	Target:	
Other Fruits	Ate:	☐☐☐☐☐☐☐☐☐☐
	Target:	
Most Dairy	Ate:	☐☐☐☐☐☐☐☐☐☐
	Target:	
Fatty Meat/Oils	Ate:	☐☐☐☐☐☐☐☐☐☐
	Target:	
Starchy Vegetables/Starch	Ate:	☐☐☐☐☐☐☐☐☐☐
	Target:	
Sweets/Sweetened Drinks	Ate:	☐☐☐☐☐☐☐☐☐☐
	Target:	

Today I am proud that I: _____
_____
_____

Today I noticed that eating more and exercising less—smarter—
had a positive impact on my life when: _____
_____
_____

What I ate today: _____

_____

_____

_____

_____

_____

_____

_____

_____

What did I do well? _____

_____

_____

_____

_____

_____

_____

_____

_____

Tomorrow I can eat more—smarter—5% more effectively by:

_____

_____

_____

_____

_____

_____

_____

Week 6—Day 3   Date:

Non-Starchy Vegetables	Ate:	☐☐☐☐☐☐☐☐☐☐☐
	Target:	■■■■■■■■■■■
Seafood/Lean Meat/Egg Whites/Whey/Select Dairy	Ate:	☐☐☐☐☐☐☐☐☐☐☐
	Target:	■■■■■
Flax Seeds/Nuts	Ate:	☐☐☐☐☐☐☐☐☐☐☐
	Target:	■■■■■
Berries/Citrus Fruits	Ate:	☐☐☐☐☐☐☐☐☐☐☐
	Target:	■■■■■
Legumes	Ate:	☐☐☐☐☐☐☐☐☐☐☐
	Target:	
Other Fruits	Ate:	☐☐☐☐☐☐☐☐☐☐☐
	Target:	
Most Dairy	Ate:	☐☐☐☐☐☐☐☐☐☐☐
	Target:	
Fatty Meat/Oils	Ate:	☐☐☐☐☐☐☐☐☐☐☐
	Target:	
Starchy Vegetables/Starch	Ate:	☐☐☐☐☐☐☐☐☐☐☐
	Target:	
Sweets/Sweetened Drinks	Ate:	☐☐☐☐☐☐☐☐☐☐☐
	Target:	

Today I am proud that I: _____

_____

_____

Today I noticed that eating more and exercising less—smarter—
had a positive impact on my life when: _____

_____

_____

_____

What I ate today: _____
_____
_____
_____
_____
_____
_____
_____
_____
_____

What did I do well? _____
_____
_____
_____
_____
_____
_____
_____
_____
_____

Tomorrow I can eat more—smarter—5% more effectively by:
_____
_____
_____
_____
_____
_____
_____
_____
_____

Week 6—Day 4   Date:

Non-Starchy Vegetables	Ate:	☐☐☐☐☐☐☐☐☐☐
	Target:	■■■■■■■■■■
Seafood/Lean Meat/Egg Whites/Whey/Select Dairy	Ate:	☐☐☐☐☐☐☐☐☐☐
	Target:	■■■■■■
Flax Seeds/Nuts	Ate:	☐☐☐☐☐☐☐☐☐☐
	Target:	■■■■■■
Berries/Citrus Fruits	Ate:	☐☐☐☐☐☐☐☐☐☐
	Target:	■■■■■■
Legumes	Ate:	☐☐☐☐☐☐☐☐☐☐
	Target:	
Other Fruits	Ate:	☐☐☐☐☐☐☐☐☐☐
	Target:	
Most Dairy	Ate:	☐☐☐☐☐☐☐☐☐☐
	Target:	
Fatty Meat/Oils	Ate:	☐☐☐☐☐☐☐☐☐☐
	Target:	
Starchy Vegetables/Starch	Ate:	☐☐☐☐☐☐☐☐☐☐
	Target:	
Sweets/Sweetened Drinks	Ate:	☐☐☐☐☐☐☐☐☐☐
	Target:	

Today I am proud that I: _____

_____

_____

Today I noticed that eating more and exercising less—smarter—
had a positive impact on my life when: _____

_____

_____

_____

What I ate today: _____

_____

_____

_____

_____

_____

_____

_____

_____

_____

What did I do well? _____

_____

_____

_____

_____

_____

_____

_____

_____

_____

Tomorrow I can eat more—smarter—5% more effectively by:

_____

_____

_____

_____

_____

_____

_____

_____

_____

Week 6—Day 5   Date:

Non-Starchy Vegetables	Ate:	☐☐☐☐☐☐☐☐☐☐
	Target:	■■■■■■■■■■
Seafood/Lean Meat/Egg Whites/Whey/Select Dairy	Ate:	☐☐☐☐☐☐☐☐☐☐
	Target:	■■■■■■
Flax Seeds/Nuts	Ate:	☐☐☐☐☐☐☐☐☐☐
	Target:	■■■■■■
Berries/Citrus Fruits	Ate:	☐☐☐☐☐☐☐☐☐☐
	Target:	■■■■■■
Legumes	Ate:	☐☐☐☐☐☐☐☐☐☐
	Target:	
Other Fruits	Ate:	☐☐☐☐☐☐☐☐☐☐
	Target:	
Most Dairy	Ate:	☐☐☐☐☐☐☐☐☐☐
	Target:	
Fatty Meat/Oils	Ate:	☐☐☐☐☐☐☐☐☐☐
	Target:	
Starchy Vegetables/Starch	Ate:	☐☐☐☐☐☐☐☐☐☐
	Target:	
Sweets/Sweetened Drinks	Ate:	☐☐☐☐☐☐☐☐☐☐
	Target:	

Today I am proud that I: _____

_____

_____

Today I noticed that eating more and exercising less—smarter—had a positive impact on my life when: _____

_____

_____

_____

What I ate today: _____
_____
_____
_____
_____
_____
_____
_____
_____
_____

What did I do well? _____
_____
_____
_____
_____
_____
_____
_____
_____
_____

Tomorrow I can eat more—smarter—5% more effectively by:
_____
_____
_____
_____
_____
_____
_____
_____
_____
_____

THE SMARTER SCIENCE OF SLIM JOURNAL

Week 6—Day 6   Date:

Non-Starchy Vegetables	Ate:	□□□□□□□□□□	
	Target:	■■■■■■■■■■	
Seafood/Lean Meat/Egg Whites/Whey/Select Dairy	Ate:	□□□□□□□□□□	
	Target:	■■■■■	
Flax Seeds/Nuts	Ate:	□□□□□□□□□□	
	Target:	■■■■■	
Berries/Citrus Fruits	Ate:	□□□□□□□□□□	
	Target:	■■■■■	
Legumes	Ate:	□□□□□□□□□□	
	Target:		
Other Fruits	Ate:	□□□□□□□□□□	
	Target:		
Most Dairy	Ate:	□□□□□□□□□□	
	Target:		
Fatty Meat/Oils	Ate:	□□□□□□□□□□	
	Target:		
Starchy Vegetables/Starch	Ate:	□□□□□□□□□□	
	Target:		
Sweets/Sweetened Drinks	Ate:	□□□□□□□□□□	
	Target:		

Today I am proud that I: _____

_____

_____

Today I noticed that eating more and exercising less—smarter—
had a positive impact on my life when: _____

_____

_____

_____

What I ate today: _____

_____

_____

_____

_____

_____

_____

_____

_____

_____

What did I do well? _____

_____

_____

_____

_____

_____

_____

_____

_____

_____

Tomorrow I can eat more—smarter—5% more effectively by:

_____

_____

_____

_____

_____

_____

_____

_____

_____

Week 6—Day 7   Date:

Non-Starchy Vegetables   Ate: ☐☐☐☐☐☐☐☐☐☐☐☐
Target: ■■■■■■■■■■■

Seafood/Lean Meat/Egg Whites/Whey/Select Dairy   Ate: ☐☐☐☐☐☐☐☐☐☐☐☐
Target: ■■■■■

Flax Seeds/Nuts   Ate: ☐☐☐☐☐☐☐☐☐☐☐☐
Target: ■■■■■

Berries/Citrus Fruits   Ate: ☐☐☐☐☐☐☐☐☐☐☐☐
Target: ■■■■■

Legumes   Ate: ☐☐☐☐☐☐☐☐☐☐☐
Target:

Other Fruits   Ate: ☐☐☐☐☐☐☐☐☐☐☐
Target:

Most Dairy   Ate: ☐☐☐☐☐☐☐☐☐☐☐
Target:

Fatty Meat/Oils   Ate: ☐☐☐☐☐☐☐☐☐☐☐
Target:

Starchy Vegetables/Starch   Ate: ☐☐☐☐☐☐☐☐☐☐☐
Target:

Sweets/Sweetened Drinks   Ate: ☐☐☐☐☐☐☐☐☐☐☐
Target:

Today I am proud that I: _____
_____
_____

Today I noticed that eating more and exercising less—smarter—had a positive impact on my life when: _____
_____
_____
_____

What I ate today: _____

_____

_____

_____

_____

_____

_____

_____

_____

What did I do well? _____

_____

_____

_____

_____

_____

_____

_____

_____

_____

Tomorrow I can eat more—smarter—5% more effectively by:

_____

_____

_____

_____

_____

_____

_____

_____

_____

Week 6 Eccentric Exercise   Date:

Home Option

		Add resistance?
Assisted Eccentric Squats	Resistance: _____	Y / N
Assisted Eccentric Pull-Ups	Resistance: _____	Y / N
Assisted Eccentric Push-Ups	Resistance: _____	Y / N
Assisted Eccentric Shoulder Press	Resistance: _____	Y / N

Gym Option

		Add resistance?
Eccentric Leg Presses	Resistance: _____	Y / N
Eccentric Rows	Resistance: _____	Y / N
Eccentric Check Presses	Resistance: _____	Y / N
Eccentric Shoulder Presses	Resistance: _____	Y / N

Week 1 Cardiovascular Exercise   Date:

		Add resistance?
10 Minutes of High-Quality Brief Cardiovascular Exercise	Resistance: _____	Y / N

Remember: It should be impossible to do more than six repetitions of each eccentric exercise per week. It should also be impossible to do more than six repetitions of brief cardiovascular exercise per week. If more repetitions are possible or more workouts are possible, then add resistance.

Notes: _____

_____

_____

_____

_____

_____

_____

_____

_____

_____

What did I do well? _____

_____

_____

_____

_____

_____

_____

_____

_____

_____

Next week I can exercise less—smarter—5% more effectively by:

_____

_____

_____

_____

_____

_____

_____

_____

Week 7—Day 1   Date:

Non-Starchy Vegetables	Ate:	☐☐☐☐☐☐☐☐☐☐
	Target:	■■■■■■■■■■
Seafood/Lean Meat/Egg Whites/Whey/Select Dairy	Ate:	☐☐☐☐☐☐☐☐☐☐
	Target:	■■■■■
Flax Seeds/Nuts	Ate:	☐☐☐☐☐☐☐☐☐☐
	Target:	■■■■■
Berries/Citrus Fruits	Ate:	☐☐☐☐☐☐☐☐☐☐
	Target:	■■■■■
Legumes	Ate:	☐☐☐☐☐☐☐☐☐☐
	Target:	
Other Fruits	Ate:	☐☐☐☐☐☐☐☐☐☐
	Target:	
Most Dairy	Ate:	☐☐☐☐☐☐☐☐☐☐
	Target:	
Fatty Meat/Oils	Ate:	☐☐☐☐☐☐☐☐☐☐
	Target:	
Starchy Vegetables/Starch	Ate:	☐☐☐☐☐☐☐☐☐☐
	Target:	
Sweets/Sweetened Drinks	Ate:	☐☐☐☐☐☐☐☐☐☐
	Target:	

Today I am proud that I: _____

_____

_____

Today I noticed that eating more and exercising less—smarter—
had a positive impact on my life when: _____

_____

_____

_____

What I ate today: _____

_____

_____

_____

_____

_____

_____

_____

_____

_____

What did I do well? _____

_____

_____

_____

_____

_____

_____

_____

_____

_____

_____

Tomorrow I can eat more—smarter—5% more effectively by:

_____

_____

_____

_____

_____

_____

_____

_____

_____

Week 7—Day 2   Date:

		Ate	Target
Non-Starchy Vegetables	Ate:	□□□□□□□□□□□	
	Target:	■■■■■■■■■■	
Seafood/Lean Meat/Egg Whites/Whey/Select Dairy	Ate:	□□□□□□□□□□□	
	Target:	■■■■■	
Flax Seeds/Nuts	Ate:	□□□□□□□□□□□	
	Target:	■■■■■	
Berries/Citrus Fruits	Ate:	□□□□□□□□□□□	
	Target:	■■■■■	
Legumes	Ate:	□□□□□□□□□□□	
	Target:		
Other Fruits	Ate:	□□□□□□□□□□□	
	Target:		
Most Dairy	Ate:	□□□□□□□□□□□	
	Target:		
Fatty Meat/Oils	Ate:	□□□□□□□□□□□	
	Target:		
Starchy Vegetables/Starch	Ate:	□□□□□□□□□□□	
	Target:		
Sweets/Sweetened Drinks	Ate:	□□□□□□□□□□□	
	Target:		

Today I am proud that I: _____

_____

_____

Today I noticed that eating more and exercising less—smarter—
had a positive impact on my life when: _____

_____

_____

_____

What I ate today: _____

_____

_____

_____

_____

_____

_____

_____

_____

_____

What did I do well? _____

_____

_____

_____

_____

_____

_____

_____

_____

_____

Tomorrow I can eat more—smarter—5% more effectively by:

_____

_____

_____

_____

_____

_____

_____

_____

_____

Week 7—Day 3   Date:

Non-Starchy Vegetables	Ate:	☐	☐	☐	☐	☐	☐	☐	☐	☐	☐	☐
	Target:	■	■	■	■	■	■	■	■	■	■	■
Seafood/Lean Meat/Egg Whites/Whey/Select Dairy	Ate:	☐	☐	☐	☐	☐	☐	☐	☐	☐	☐	☐
	Target:	■	■	■	■	■						
Flax Seeds/Nuts	Ate:	☐	☐	☐	☐	☐	☐	☐	☐	☐	☐	☐
	Target:	■	■	■	■	■						
Berries/Citrus Fruits	Ate:	☐	☐	☐	☐	☐	☐	☐	☐	☐	☐	☐
	Target:	■	■	■	■	■						
Legumes	Ate:	☐	☐	☐	☐	☐	☐	☐	☐	☐	☐	☐
	Target:											
Other Fruits	Ate:	☐	☐	☐	☐	☐	☐	☐	☐	☐	☐	☐
	Target:											
Most Dairy	Ate:	☐	☐	☐	☐	☐	☐	☐	☐	☐	☐	☐
	Target:											
Fatty Meat/Oils	Ate:	☐	☐	☐	☐	☐	☐	☐	☐	☐	☐	☐
	Target:											
Starchy Vegetables/Starch	Ate:	☐	☐	☐	☐	☐	☐	☐	☐	☐	☐	☐
	Target:											
Sweets/Sweetened Drinks	Ate:	☐	☐	☐	☐	☐	☐	☐	☐	☐	☐	☐
	Target:											

Today I am proud that I: _____

_____

_____

Today I noticed that eating more and exercising less—smarter—
had a positive impact on my life when: _____

_____

_____

_____

What I ate today: _____
_____
_____
_____
_____
_____
_____
_____
_____
_____
_____

What did I do well? _____
_____
_____
_____
_____
_____
_____
_____
_____
_____
_____

Tomorrow I can eat more—smarter—5% more effectively by:
_____
_____
_____
_____
_____
_____
_____
_____
_____

Week 7—Day 4   Date:

Non-Starchy Vegetables	Ate:	☐☐☐☐☐☐☐☐☐☐
	Target:	■■■■■■■■■■
Seafood/Lean Meat/Egg Whites/Whey/Select Dairy	Ate:	☐☐☐☐☐☐☐☐☐☐
	Target:	■■■■■
Flax Seeds/Nuts	Ate:	☐☐☐☐☐☐☐☐☐☐
	Target:	■■■■■
Berries/Citrus Fruits	Ate:	☐☐☐☐☐☐☐☐☐☐
	Target:	■■■■■
Legumes	Ate:	☐☐☐☐☐☐☐☐☐☐
	Target:	
Other Fruits	Ate:	☐☐☐☐☐☐☐☐☐☐
	Target:	
Most Dairy	Ate:	☐☐☐☐☐☐☐☐☐☐
	Target:	
Fatty Meat/Oils	Ate:	☐☐☐☐☐☐☐☐☐☐
	Target:	
Starchy Vegetables/Starch	Ate:	☐☐☐☐☐☐☐☐☐☐
	Target:	
Sweets/Sweetened Drinks	Ate:	☐☐☐☐☐☐☐☐☐☐
	Target:	

Today I am proud that I: _____

_____

_____

Today I noticed that eating more and exercising less—smarter—
had a positive impact on my life when: _____

_____

_____

_____

What I ate today: _____
_____
_____
_____
_____
_____
_____
_____
_____

What did I do well? _____
_____
_____
_____
_____
_____
_____
_____
_____
_____

Tomorrow I can eat more—smarter—5% more effectively by:
_____
_____
_____
_____
_____
_____
_____
_____
_____

Week 7—Day 5   Date:

Non-Starchy Vegetables	Ate:	☐☐☐☐☐☐☐☐☐☐☐
	Target:	■■■■■■■■■■■
Seafood/Lean Meat/Egg Whites/Whey/Select Dairy	Ate:	☐☐☐☐☐☐☐☐☐☐☐
	Target:	■■■■■
Flax Seeds/Nuts	Ate:	☐☐☐☐☐☐☐☐☐☐☐
	Target:	■■■■■
Berries/Citrus Fruits	Ate:	☐☐☐☐☐☐☐☐☐☐☐
	Target:	■■■■■
Legumes	Ate:	☐☐☐☐☐☐☐☐☐☐☐
	Target:	
Other Fruits	Ate:	☐☐☐☐☐☐☐☐☐☐
	Target:	
Most Dairy	Ate:	☐☐☐☐☐☐☐☐☐☐
	Target:	
Fatty Meat/Oils	Ate:	☐☐☐☐☐☐☐☐☐☐
	Target:	
Starchy Vegetables/Starch	Ate:	☐☐☐☐☐☐☐☐☐☐
	Target:	
Sweets/Sweetened Drinks	Ate:	☐☐☐☐☐☐☐☐☐☐
	Target:	

Today I am proud that I: _____

_____

_____

Today I noticed that eating more and exercising less—smarter—
had a positive impact on my life when: _____

_____

_____

_____

What I ate today: _____
_____
_____
_____
_____
_____
_____
_____
_____
_____

What did I do well? _____
_____
_____
_____
_____
_____
_____
_____
_____
_____
_____

Tomorrow I can eat more—smarter—5% more effectively by:
_____
_____
_____
_____
_____
_____
_____
_____
_____
_____

Week 7—Day 6   Date:

Non-Starchy Vegetables	Ate:	☐☐☐☐☐☐☐☐☐☐
	Target:	■■■■■■■■■■
Seafood/Lean Meat/Egg Whites/Whey/Select Dairy	Ate:	☐☐☐☐☐☐☐☐☐☐
	Target:	■■■■■
Flax Seeds/Nuts	Ate:	☐☐☐☐☐☐☐☐☐☐
	Target:	■■■■■
Berries/Citrus Fruits	Ate:	☐☐☐☐☐☐☐☐☐☐
	Target:	■■■■■
Legumes	Ate:	☐☐☐☐☐☐☐☐☐☐
	Target:	
Other Fruits	Ate:	☐☐☐☐☐☐☐☐☐☐
	Target:	
Most Dairy	Ate:	☐☐☐☐☐☐☐☐☐☐
	Target:	
Fatty Meat/Oils	Ate:	☐☐☐☐☐☐☐☐☐☐
	Target:	
Starchy Vegetables/Starch	Ate:	☐☐☐☐☐☐☐☐☐☐
	Target:	
Sweets/Sweetened Drinks	Ate:	☐☐☐☐☐☐☐☐☐☐
	Target:	

Today I am proud that I: _____

_____

_____

Today I noticed that eating more and exercising less—smarter—had a positive impact on my life when: _____

_____

_____

_____

What I ate today: _____

_____

_____

_____

_____

_____

_____

_____

_____

What did I do well? _____

_____

_____

_____

_____

_____

_____

_____

_____

_____

Tomorrow I can eat more—smarter—5% more effectively by:

_____

_____

_____

_____

_____

_____

_____

_____

_____

Week 7—Day 7   Date:

Non-Starchy Vegetables	Ate:	☐☐☐☐☐☐☐☐☐☐☐
	Target:	■■■■■■■■■■
Seafood/Lean Meat/Egg Whites/Whey/Select Dairy	Ate:	☐☐☐☐☐☐☐☐☐☐☐
	Target:	■■■■■
Flax Seeds/Nuts	Ate:	☐☐☐☐☐☐☐☐☐☐☐
	Target:	■■■■■
Berries/Citrus Fruits	Ate:	☐☐☐☐☐☐☐☐☐☐☐
	Target:	■■■■■
Legumes	Ate:	☐☐☐☐☐☐☐☐☐☐☐
	Target:	
Other Fruits	Ate:	☐☐☐☐☐☐☐☐☐☐☐
	Target:	
Most Dairy	Ate:	☐☐☐☐☐☐☐☐☐☐☐
	Target:	
Fatty Meat/Oils	Ate:	☐☐☐☐☐☐☐☐☐☐☐
	Target:	
Starchy Vegetables/Starch	Ate:	☐☐☐☐☐☐☐☐☐☐☐
	Target:	
Sweets/Sweetened Drinks	Ate:	☐☐☐☐☐☐☐☐☐☐☐
	Target:	

Today I am proud that I: _____

_____

_____

Today I noticed that eating more and exercising less—smarter—
had a positive impact on my life when: _____

_____

_____

_____

What I ate today: _____

_____

_____

_____

_____

_____

_____

_____

_____

_____

What did I do well? _____

_____

_____

_____

_____

_____

_____

_____

_____

_____

_____

Tomorrow I can eat more—smarter—5% more effectively by:

_____

_____

_____

_____

_____

_____

_____

_____

_____

_____

Week 7 Eccentric Exercise   Date:

Home Option

		Add resistance?
Assisted Eccentric Squats	Resistance: _____	Y / N
Assisted Eccentric Pull-Ups	Resistance: _____	Y / N
Assisted Eccentric Push-Ups	Resistance: _____	Y / N
Assisted Eccentric Shoulder Press	Resistance: _____	Y / N

Gym Option

		Add resistance?
Eccentric Leg Presses	Resistance: _____	Y / N
Eccentric Rows	Resistance: _____	Y / N
Eccentric Check Presses	Resistance: _____	Y / N
Eccentric Shoulder Presses	Resistance: _____	Y / N

Week 1 Cardiovascular Exercise   Date:

		Add resistance?
10 Minutes of High-Quality Brief Cardiovascular Exercise	Resistance: _____	Y / N

Remember: It should be impossible to do more than six repetitions of each eccentric exercise per week. It should also be impossible to do more than six repetitions of brief cardiovascular exercise per week. If more repetitions are possible or more workouts are possible, then add resistance.

Notes: _____
_____
_____
_____
_____
_____
_____
_____
_____
_____
_____
_____

What did I do well? _____
_____
_____
_____
_____
_____
_____
_____
_____
_____
_____
_____

Next week I can exercise less—smarter—5% more effectively by:
_____
_____
_____
_____
_____
_____
_____
_____
_____
_____
_____

Week 8—Day 1   Date:

Non-Starchy Vegetables	Ate:	☐☐☐☐☐☐☐☐☐☐☐
	Target:	■■■■■■■■■■
Seafood/Lean Meat/Egg Whites/Whey/Select Dairy	Ate:	☐☐☐☐☐☐☐☐☐☐☐
	Target:	■■■■■
Flax Seeds/Nuts	Ate:	☐☐☐☐☐☐☐☐☐☐☐
	Target:	■■■■■
Berries/Citrus Fruits	Ate:	☐☐☐☐☐☐☐☐☐☐☐
	Target:	■■■■■
Legumes	Ate:	☐☐☐☐☐☐☐☐☐☐☐
	Target:	
Other Fruits	Ate:	☐☐☐☐☐☐☐☐☐☐☐
	Target:	
Most Dairy	Ate:	☐☐☐☐☐☐☐☐☐☐☐
	Target:	
Fatty Meat/Oils	Ate:	☐☐☐☐☐☐☐☐☐☐☐
	Target:	
Starchy Vegetables/Starch	Ate:	☐☐☐☐☐☐☐☐☐☐☐
	Target:	
Sweets/Sweetened Drinks	Ate:	☐☐☐☐☐☐☐☐☐☐
	Target:	

Today I am proud that I: _____

_____

_____

Today I noticed that eating more and exercising less—smarter—had a positive impact on my life when: _____

_____

_____

_____

What I ate today: _____
_____
_____
_____
_____
_____
_____
_____
_____
_____

What did I do well? _____
_____
_____
_____
_____
_____
_____
_____
_____
_____

Tomorrow I can eat more—smarter—5% more effectively by:
_____
_____
_____
_____
_____
_____
_____
_____
_____

Week 8—Day 2   Date:

		Ate:	Target:
Non-Starchy Vegetables	Ate:	□□□□□□□□□□	
	Target:	■■■■■■■■■■	
Seafood/Lean Meat/Egg Whites/Whey/Select Dairy	Ate:	□□□□□□□□□□	
	Target:	■■■■■	
Flax Seeds/Nuts	Ate:	□□□□□□□□□□	
	Target:	■■■■■	
Berries/Citrus Fruits	Ate:	□□□□□□□□□□	
	Target:	■■■■■	
Legumes	Ate:	□□□□□□□□□□	
	Target:		
Other Fruits	Ate:	□□□□□□□□□□	
	Target:		
Most Dairy	Ate:	□□□□□□□□□□	
	Target:		
Fatty Meat/Oils	Ate:	□□□□□□□□□□	
	Target:		
Starchy Vegetables/Starch	Ate:	□□□□□□□□□□	
	Target:		
Sweets/Sweetened Drinks	Ate:	□□□□□□□□□□	
	Target:		

Today I am proud that I: _____

_____

_____

Today I noticed that eating more and exercising less—smarter—
had a positive impact on my life when: _____

_____

_____

_____

What I ate today: _____
_____
_____
_____
_____
_____
_____
_____
_____
_____

What did I do well? _____
_____
_____
_____
_____
_____
_____
_____
_____
_____
_____

Tomorrow I can eat more—smarter—5% more effectively by:
_____
_____
_____
_____
_____
_____
_____
_____
_____

Week 8—Day 3   Date:

Non-Starchy Vegetables	Ate:	☐☐☐☐☐☐☐☐☐☐☐☐
	Target:	■■■■■■■■■■■■
Seafood/Lean Meat/Egg Whites/Whey/Select Dairy	Ate:	☐☐☐☐☐☐☐☐☐☐☐☐
	Target:	■■■■■
Flax Seeds/Nuts	Ate:	☐☐☐☐☐☐☐☐☐☐☐☐
	Target:	■■■■■
Berries/Citrus Fruits	Ate:	☐☐☐☐☐☐☐☐☐☐☐☐
	Target:	■■■■■
Legumes	Ate:	☐☐☐☐☐☐☐☐☐☐☐☐
	Target:	
Other Fruits	Ate:	☐☐☐☐☐☐☐☐☐☐☐☐
	Target:	
Most Dairy	Ate:	☐☐☐☐☐☐☐☐☐☐☐☐
	Target:	
Fatty Meat/Oils	Ate:	☐☐☐☐☐☐☐☐☐☐☐☐
	Target:	
Starchy Vegetables/Starch	Ate:	☐☐☐☐☐☐☐☐☐☐☐☐
	Target:	
Sweets/Sweetened Drinks	Ate:	☐☐☐☐☐☐☐☐☐☐☐
	Target:	

Today I am proud that I: _____

_____

_____

Today I noticed that eating more and exercising less—smarter—
had a positive impact on my life when: _____

_____

_____

_____

What I ate today: _____

_____

_____

_____

_____

_____

_____

_____

_____

_____

What did I do well? _____

_____

_____

_____

_____

_____

_____

_____

_____

_____

Tomorrow I can eat more—smarter—5% more effectively by:

_____

_____

_____

_____

_____

_____

_____

_____

_____

Week 8—Day 4   Date:

Non-Starchy Vegetables Ate: ☐☐☐☐☐☐☐☐☐☐
Target: ■■■■■■■■■■

Seafood/Lean Meat/Egg Whites/Whey/Select Dairy Ate: ☐☐☐☐☐☐☐☐☐☐
Target: ■■■■■

Flax Seeds/Nuts Ate: ☐☐☐☐☐☐☐☐☐☐
Target: ■■■■■

Berries/Citrus Fruits Ate: ☐☐☐☐☐☐☐☐☐☐
Target: ■■■■■

Legumes Ate: ☐☐☐☐☐☐☐☐☐☐
Target:

Other Fruits Ate: ☐☐☐☐☐☐☐☐☐☐
Target:

Most Dairy Ate: ☐☐☐☐☐☐☐☐☐☐
Target:

Fatty Meat/Oils Ate: ☐☐☐☐☐☐☐☐☐☐
Target:

Starchy Vegetables/Starch Ate: ☐☐☐☐☐☐☐☐☐☐
Target:

Sweets/Sweetened Drinks Ate: ☐☐☐☐☐☐☐☐☐☐
Target:

Today I am proud that I: _____
_____
_____

Today I noticed that eating more and exercising less—smarter—had a positive impact on my life when: _____
_____
_____
_____

What I ate today: _____

_____

_____

_____

_____

_____

_____

_____

_____

_____

What did I do well? _____

_____

_____

_____

_____

_____

_____

_____

_____

_____

_____

Tomorrow I can eat more—smarter—5% more effectively by:

_____

_____

_____

_____

_____

_____

_____

_____

_____

Week 8—Day 5   Date:

Non-Starchy Vegetables	Ate:	☐☐☐☐☐☐☐☐☐☐☐
	Target:	■■■■■■■■■■
Seafood/Lean Meat/Egg Whites/Whey/Select Dairy	Ate:	☐☐☐☐☐☐☐☐☐☐☐
	Target:	■■■■■
Flax Seeds/Nuts	Ate:	☐☐☐☐☐☐☐☐☐☐☐
	Target:	■■■■■
Berries/Citrus Fruits	Ate:	☐☐☐☐☐☐☐☐☐☐☐
	Target:	■■■■■
Legumes	Ate:	☐☐☐☐☐☐☐☐☐☐☐
	Target:	
Other Fruits	Ate:	☐☐☐☐☐☐☐☐☐☐☐
	Target:	
Most Dairy	Ate:	☐☐☐☐☐☐☐☐☐☐☐
	Target:	
Fatty Meat/Oils	Ate:	☐☐☐☐☐☐☐☐☐☐☐
	Target:	
Starchy Vegetables/Starch	Ate:	☐☐☐☐☐☐☐☐☐☐☐
	Target:	
Sweets/Sweetened Drinks	Ate:	☐☐☐☐☐☐☐☐☐☐☐
	Target:	

Today I am proud that I: _____

_____

_____

Today I noticed that eating more and exercising less—smarter—
had a positive impact on my life when: _____

_____

_____

_____

What I ate today: _____
_____
_____
_____
_____
_____
_____
_____
_____
_____

What did I do well? _____
_____
_____
_____
_____
_____
_____
_____
_____
_____
_____

Tomorrow I can eat more—smarter—5% more effectively by:
_____
_____
_____
_____
_____
_____
_____
_____
_____

Week 8—Day 6   Date:

Non-Starchy Vegetables	Ate:	☐☐☐☐☐☐☐☐☐☐☐
	Target:	■■■■■■■■■■
Seafood/Lean Meat/Egg Whites/Whey/Select Dairy	Ate:	☐☐☐☐☐☐☐☐☐☐
	Target:	■■■■■
Flax Seeds/Nuts	Ate:	☐☐☐☐☐☐☐☐☐☐
	Target:	■■■■■
Berries/Citrus Fruits	Ate:	☐☐☐☐☐☐☐☐☐☐
	Target:	■■■■■
Legumes	Ate:	☐☐☐☐☐☐☐☐☐☐
	Target:	
Other Fruits	Ate:	☐☐☐☐☐☐☐☐☐☐
	Target:	
Most Dairy	Ate:	☐☐☐☐☐☐☐☐☐☐
	Target:	
Fatty Meat/Oils	Ate:	☐☐☐☐☐☐☐☐☐☐
	Target:	
Starchy Vegetables/Starch	Ate:	☐☐☐☐☐☐☐☐☐☐
	Target:	
Sweets/Sweetened Drinks	Ate:	☐☐☐☐☐☐☐☐☐☐
	Target:	

Today I am proud that I: _____

_____

_____

Today I noticed that eating more and exercising less—smarter—
had a positive impact on my life when: _____

_____

_____

_____

What I ate today: _____
_____
_____
_____
_____
_____
_____
_____
_____
_____
_____

What did I do well? _____
_____
_____
_____
_____
_____
_____
_____
_____
_____
_____
_____

Tomorrow I can eat more—smarter—5% more effectively by:
_____
_____
_____
_____
_____
_____
_____
_____
_____

Week 8—Day 7   Date:

		Ate:	☐☐☐☐☐☐☐☐☐☐☐
Non-Starchy Vegetables		Target:	■■■■■■■■■■■
Seafood/Lean Meat/Egg Whites/Whey/Select Dairy		Ate:	☐☐☐☐☐☐☐☐☐☐☐
		Target:	■■■■■
Flax Seeds/Nuts		Ate:	☐☐☐☐☐☐☐☐☐☐☐
		Target:	■■■■■
Berries/Citrus Fruits		Ate:	☐☐☐☐☐☐☐☐☐☐☐
		Target:	■■■■■
Legumes		Ate:	☐☐☐☐☐☐☐☐☐☐☐
		Target:	
Other Fruits		Ate:	☐☐☐☐☐☐☐☐☐☐☐
		Target:	
Most Dairy		Ate:	☐☐☐☐☐☐☐☐☐☐☐
		Target:	
Fatty Meat/Oils		Ate:	☐☐☐☐☐☐☐☐☐☐☐
		Target:	
Starchy Vegetables/Starch		Ate:	☐☐☐☐☐☐☐☐☐☐☐
		Target:	
Sweets/Sweetened Drinks		Ate:	☐☐☐☐☐☐☐☐☐☐☐
		Target:	

Today I am proud that I: _____

_____

_____

Today I noticed that eating more and exercising less—smarter—
had a positive impact on my life when: _____

_____

_____

_____

What I ate today: _____

_____

_____

_____

_____

_____

_____

_____

_____

_____

What did I do well? _____

_____

_____

_____

_____

_____

_____

_____

_____

_____

Tomorrow I can eat more—smarter—5% more effectively by:

_____

_____

_____

_____

_____

_____

_____

_____

_____

Week 8 Eccentric Exercise   Date:

Home Option

		Add resistance?
Assisted Eccentric Squats	Resistance: _____	Y / N
Assisted Eccentric Pull-Ups	Resistance: _____	Y / N
Assisted Eccentric Push-Ups	Resistance: _____	Y / N
Assisted Eccentric Shoulder Press	Resistance: _____	Y / N

Gym Option

		Add resistance?
Eccentric Leg Presses	Resistance: _____	Y / N
Eccentric Rows	Resistance: _____	Y / N
Eccentric Check Presses	Resistance: _____	Y / N
Eccentric Shoulder Presses	Resistance: _____	Y / N

Week 1 Cardiovascular Exercise   Date:

		Add resistance?
10 Minutes of High-Quality Brief Cardiovascular Exercise	Resistance: _____	Y / N

Remember: It should be impossible to do more than six repetitions of each eccentric exercise per week. It should also be impossible to do more than six repetitions of brief cardiovascular exercise per week. If more repetitions are possible or more workouts are possible, then add resistance.

Notes: _____

_____

_____

_____

_____

_____

_____

_____

_____

_____

_____

What did I do well? _____

_____

_____

_____

_____

_____

_____

_____

_____

_____

_____

Next week I can exercise less—smarter—5% more effectively by:

_____

_____

_____

_____

_____

_____

_____

_____

_____

Week 9—Day 1   Date:

Non-Starchy Vegetables	Ate:	☐☐☐☐☐☐☐☐☐☐
	Target:	■■■■■■■■■■
Seafood/Lean Meat/Egg Whites/Whey/Select Dairy	Ate:	☐☐☐☐☐☐☐☐☐☐
	Target:	■■■■■
Flax Seeds/Nuts	Ate:	☐☐☐☐☐☐☐☐☐☐
	Target:	■■■■■
Berries/Citrus Fruits	Ate:	☐☐☐☐☐☐☐☐☐☐
	Target:	■■■■■
Legumes	Ate:	☐☐☐☐☐☐☐☐☐☐
	Target:	
Other Fruits	Ate:	☐☐☐☐☐☐☐☐☐☐
	Target:	
Most Dairy	Ate:	☐☐☐☐☐☐☐☐☐☐
	Target:	
Fatty Meat/Oils	Ate:	☐☐☐☐☐☐☐☐☐☐
	Target:	
Starchy Vegetables/Starch	Ate:	☐☐☐☐☐☐☐☐☐☐
	Target:	
Sweets/Sweetened Drinks	Ate:	☐☐☐☐☐☐☐☐☐☐
	Target:	

Today I am proud that I: _____

_____

_____

Today I noticed that eating more and exercising less—smarter—had a positive impact on my life when: _____

_____

_____

_____

What I ate today: _____

_____

_____

_____

_____

_____

_____

_____

_____

_____

What did I do well? _____

_____

_____

_____

_____

_____

_____

_____

_____

_____

Tomorrow I can eat more—smarter—5% more effectively by:

_____

_____

_____

_____

_____

_____

_____

_____

_____

_____

Week 9—Day 2   Date:

Non-Starchy Vegetables	Ate:	☐☐☐☐☐☐☐☐☐☐
	Target:	■■■■■■■■■■
Seafood/Lean Meat/Egg Whites/Whey/Select Dairy	Ate:	☐☐☐☐☐☐☐☐☐☐
	Target:	■■■■■
Flax Seeds/Nuts	Ate:	☐☐☐☐☐☐☐☐☐☐
	Target:	■■■■■
Berries/Citrus Fruits	Ate:	☐☐☐☐☐☐☐☐☐☐
	Target:	■■■■■
Legumes	Ate:	☐☐☐☐☐☐☐☐☐☐
	Target:	
Other Fruits	Ate:	☐☐☐☐☐☐☐☐☐☐
	Target:	
Most Dairy	Ate:	☐☐☐☐☐☐☐☐☐☐
	Target:	
Fatty Meat/Oils	Ate:	☐☐☐☐☐☐☐☐☐☐
	Target:	
Starchy Vegetables/Starch	Ate:	☐☐☐☐☐☐☐☐☐☐
	Target:	
Sweets/Sweetened Drinks	Ate:	☐☐☐☐☐☐☐☐☐☐
	Target:	

Today I am proud that I: _____

_____

_____

Today I noticed that eating more and exercising less—smarter—
had a positive impact on my life when: _____

_____

_____

_____

What I ate today: _____

_____

_____

_____

_____

_____

_____

_____

_____

_____

_____

What did I do well? _____

_____

_____

_____

_____

_____

_____

_____

_____

_____

_____

Tomorrow I can eat more—smarter—5% more effectively by:

_____

_____

_____

_____

_____

_____

_____

_____

_____

_____

Week 9—Day 3   Date:

Non-Starchy Vegetables	Ate:	☐☐☐☐☐☐☐☐☐☐☐☐
	Target:	■■■■■■■■■■
Seafood/Lean Meat/Egg Whites/Whey/Select Dairy	Ate:	☐☐☐☐☐☐☐☐☐☐☐☐
	Target:	■■■■■
Flax Seeds/Nuts	Ate:	☐☐☐☐☐☐☐☐☐☐☐☐
	Target:	■■■■■
Berries/Citrus Fruits	Ate:	☐☐☐☐☐☐☐☐☐☐☐☐
	Target:	■■■■■
Legumes	Ate:	☐☐☐☐☐☐☐☐☐☐☐☐
	Target:	
Other Fruits	Ate:	☐☐☐☐☐☐☐☐☐☐☐☐
	Target:	
Most Dairy	Ate:	☐☐☐☐☐☐☐☐☐☐☐☐
	Target:	
Fatty Meat/Oils	Ate:	☐☐☐☐☐☐☐☐☐☐☐☐
	Target:	
Starchy Vegetables/Starch	Ate:	☐☐☐☐☐☐☐☐☐☐☐☐
	Target:	
Sweets/Sweetened Drinks	Ate:	☐☐☐☐☐☐☐☐☐☐☐☐
	Target:	

Today I am proud that I: _____

_____

_____

Today I noticed that eating more and exercising less—smarter—had a positive impact on my life when: _____

_____

_____

_____

What I ate today: _____
_____
_____
_____
_____
_____
_____
_____
_____
_____

What did I do well? _____
_____
_____
_____
_____
_____
_____
_____
_____
_____
_____

Tomorrow I can eat more—smarter—5% more effectively by:
_____
_____
_____
_____
_____
_____
_____
_____
_____
_____

Week 9—Day 4   Date:

Food		Ate	Target

Non-Starchy Vegetables
Ate: ☐☐☐☐☐☐☐☐☐☐☐
Target: ■■■■■■■■■■

Seafood/Lean Meat/Egg Whites/Whey/Select Dairy
Ate: ☐☐☐☐☐☐☐☐☐☐☐
Target: ■■■■■

Flax Seeds/Nuts
Ate: ☐☐☐☐☐☐☐☐☐☐☐
Target: ■■■■■

Berries/Citrus Fruits
Ate: ☐☐☐☐☐☐☐☐☐☐☐
Target: ■■■■■

Legumes
Ate: ☐☐☐☐☐☐☐☐☐☐☐
Target:

Other Fruits
Ate: ☐☐☐☐☐☐☐☐☐☐☐
Target:

Most Dairy
Ate: ☐☐☐☐☐☐☐☐☐☐☐
Target:

Fatty Meat/Oils
Ate: ☐☐☐☐☐☐☐☐☐☐☐
Target:

Starchy Vegetables/Starch
Ate: ☐☐☐☐☐☐☐☐☐☐☐
Target:

Sweets/Sweetened Drinks
Ate: ☐☐☐☐☐☐☐☐☐☐☐
Target:

Today I am proud that I: _____
_____
_____

Today I noticed that eating more and exercising less—smarter—had a positive impact on my life when: _____
_____
_____
_____

What I ate today: _____
_____
_____
_____
_____
_____
_____
_____
_____
_____

What did I do well? _____
_____
_____
_____
_____
_____
_____
_____
_____
_____

Tomorrow I can eat more—smarter—5% more effectively by:
_____
_____
_____
_____
_____
_____
_____
_____
_____

Week 9—Day 5   Date:

Non-Starchy Vegetables	Ate:	☐☐☐☐☐☐☐☐☐☐☐
	Target:	■■■■■■■■■■
Seafood/Lean Meat/Egg Whites/Whey/Select Dairy	Ate:	☐☐☐☐☐☐☐☐☐☐☐
	Target:	■■■■■
Flax Seeds/Nuts	Ate:	☐☐☐☐☐☐☐☐☐☐☐
	Target:	■■■■■
Berries/Citrus Fruits	Ate:	☐☐☐☐☐☐☐☐☐☐☐
	Target:	■■■■■
Legumes	Ate:	☐☐☐☐☐☐☐☐☐☐
	Target:	
Other Fruits	Ate:	☐☐☐☐☐☐☐☐☐☐
	Target:	
Most Dairy	Ate:	☐☐☐☐☐☐☐☐☐☐
	Target:	
Fatty Meat/Oils	Ate:	☐☐☐☐☐☐☐☐☐☐
	Target:	
Starchy Vegetables/Starch	Ate:	☐☐☐☐☐☐☐☐☐☐
	Target:	
Sweets/Sweetened Drinks	Ate:	☐☐☐☐☐☐☐☐☐☐
	Target:	

Today I am proud that I: _____

_____

_____

Today I noticed that eating more and exercising less—smarter—had a positive impact on my life when: _____

_____

_____

_____

What I ate today: _____

_____

_____

_____

_____

_____

_____

_____

_____

_____

What did I do well? _____

_____

_____

_____

_____

_____

_____

_____

_____

_____

Tomorrow I can eat more—smarter—5% more effectively by:

_____

_____

_____

_____

_____

_____

_____

_____

_____

Week 9—Day 6   Date:

		Ate:	Target:
Non-Starchy Vegetables	Ate:	□□□□□□□□□□	
	Target:	■■■■■■■■■■	
Seafood/Lean Meat/Egg Whites/Whey/Select Dairy	Ate:	□□□□□□□□□□	
	Target:	■■■■■	
Flax Seeds/Nuts	Ate:	□□□□□□□□□□	
	Target:	■■■■■	
Berries/Citrus Fruits	Ate:	□□□□□□□□□□	
	Target:	■■■■■	
Legumes	Ate:	□□□□□□□□□□	
	Target:		
Other Fruits	Ate:	□□□□□□□□□□	
	Target:		
Most Dairy	Ate:	□□□□□□□□□□	
	Target:		
Fatty Meat/Oils	Ate:	□□□□□□□□□□	
	Target:		
Starchy Vegetables/Starch	Ate:	□□□□□□□□□□	
	Target:		
Sweets/Sweetened Drinks	Ate:	□□□□□□□□□□	
	Target:		

Today I am proud that I: _____

_____

_____

Today I noticed that eating more and exercising less—smarter—had a positive impact on my life when: _____

_____

_____

_____

What I ate today: _____
_____
_____
_____
_____
_____
_____
_____
_____
_____
_____

What did I do well? _____
_____
_____
_____
_____
_____
_____
_____
_____
_____
_____

Tomorrow I can eat more—smarter—5% more effectively by:
_____
_____
_____
_____
_____
_____
_____
_____
_____
_____

Week 9—Day 7   Date:

Non-Starchy Vegetables	Ate:	☐☐☐☐☐☐☐☐☐☐☐
	Target:	■■■■■■■■■■
Seafood/Lean Meat/Egg Whites/Whey/Select Dairy	Ate:	☐☐☐☐☐☐☐☐☐☐☐
	Target:	■■■■■■
Flax Seeds/Nuts	Ate:	☐☐☐☐☐☐☐☐☐☐☐
	Target:	■■■■■■
Berries/Citrus Fruits	Ate:	☐☐☐☐☐☐☐☐☐☐☐
	Target:	■■■■■■
Legumes	Ate:	☐☐☐☐☐☐☐☐☐☐☐
	Target:	
Other Fruits	Ate:	☐☐☐☐☐☐☐☐☐☐☐
	Target:	
Most Dairy	Ate:	☐☐☐☐☐☐☐☐☐☐☐
	Target:	
Fatty Meat/Oils	Ate:	☐☐☐☐☐☐☐☐☐☐☐
	Target:	
Starchy Vegetables/Starch	Ate:	☐☐☐☐☐☐☐☐☐☐☐
	Target:	
Sweets/Sweetened Drinks	Ate:	☐☐☐☐☐☐☐☐☐☐☐
	Target:	

Today I am proud that I: _____

_____

_____

Today I noticed that eating more and exercising less—smarter—
had a positive impact on my life when: _____

_____

_____

_____

What I ate today: _____

_____

_____

_____

_____

_____

_____

_____

_____

_____

What did I do well? _____

_____

_____

_____

_____

_____

_____

_____

_____

_____

_____

Tomorrow I can eat more—smarter—5% more effectively by:

_____

_____

_____

_____

_____

_____

_____

_____

_____

_____

Week 9 Eccentric Exercise   Date:

Home Option

		Add resistance?
Assisted Eccentric Squats	Resistance: _____	Y / N
Assisted Eccentric Pull-Ups	Resistance: _____	Y / N
Assisted Eccentric Push-Ups	Resistance: _____	Y / N
Assisted Eccentric Shoulder Press	Resistance: _____	Y / N

Gym Option

		Add resistance?
Eccentric Leg Presses	Resistance: _____	Y / N
Eccentric Rows	Resistance: _____	Y / N
Eccentric Check Presses	Resistance: _____	Y / N
Eccentric Shoulder Presses	Resistance: _____	Y / N

Week 1 Cardiovascular Exercise   Date:

		Add resistance?
10 Minutes of High-Quality Brief Cardiovascular Exercise	Resistance: _____	Y / N

Remember: It should be impossible to do more than six repetitions of each eccentric exercise per week. It should also be impossible to do more than six repetitions of brief cardiovascular exercise per week. If more repetitions are possible or more workouts are possible, then add resistance.

Notes: _____

_____

_____

_____

_____

_____

_____

_____

_____

_____

_____

What did I do well? _____

_____

_____

_____

_____

_____

_____

_____

_____

_____

_____

Next week I can exercise less—smarter—5% more effectively by:

_____

_____

_____

_____

_____

_____

_____

_____

_____

Week 10—Day 1   Date:

Non-Starchy Vegetables	Ate:	☐☐☐☐☐☐☐☐☐☐
	Target:	■■■■■■■■■
Seafood/Lean Meat/Egg Whites/Whey/Select Dairy	Ate:	☐☐☐☐☐☐☐☐☐☐
	Target:	■■■■■
Flax Seeds/Nuts	Ate:	☐☐☐☐☐☐☐☐☐☐
	Target:	■■■■■
Berries/Citrus Fruits	Ate:	☐☐☐☐☐☐☐☐☐☐
	Target:	■■■■■
Legumes	Ate:	☐☐☐☐☐☐☐☐☐☐
	Target:	
Other Fruits	Ate:	☐☐☐☐☐☐☐☐☐☐
	Target:	
Most Dairy	Ate:	☐☐☐☐☐☐☐☐☐☐
	Target:	
Fatty Meat/Oils	Ate:	☐☐☐☐☐☐☐☐☐☐
	Target:	
Starchy Vegetables/Starch	Ate:	☐☐☐☐☐☐☐☐☐☐
	Target:	
Sweets/Sweetened Drinks	Ate:	☐☐☐☐☐☐☐☐☐☐
	Target:	

Today I am proud that I: _____

_____

_____

Today I noticed that eating more and exercising less—smarter—
had a positive impact on my life when: _____

_____

_____

What I ate today: _____
_____
_____
_____
_____
_____
_____
_____
_____
_____
_____

What did I do well? _____
_____
_____
_____
_____
_____
_____
_____
_____
_____
_____

Tomorrow I can eat more—smarter—5% more effectively by:
_____
_____
_____
_____
_____
_____
_____
_____
_____
_____

Week 10—Day 2   Date:

Non-Starchy Vegetables	Ate:	☐☐☐☐☐☐☐☐☐☐☐
	Target:	■■■■■■■■■■
Seafood/Lean Meat/Egg Whites/Whey/Select Dairy	Ate:	☐☐☐☐☐☐☐☐☐☐☐
	Target:	■■■■■
Flax Seeds/Nuts	Ate:	☐☐☐☐☐☐☐☐☐☐☐
	Target:	■■■■■
Berries/Citrus Fruits	Ate:	☐☐☐☐☐☐☐☐☐☐☐
	Target:	■■■■■
Legumes	Ate:	☐☐☐☐☐☐☐☐☐☐
	Target:	
Other Fruits	Ate:	☐☐☐☐☐☐☐☐☐☐
	Target:	
Most Dairy	Ate:	☐☐☐☐☐☐☐☐☐☐
	Target:	
Fatty Meat/Oils	Ate:	☐☐☐☐☐☐☐☐☐☐
	Target:	
Starchy Vegetables/Starch	Ate:	☐☐☐☐☐☐☐☐☐☐
	Target:	
Sweets/Sweetened Drinks	Ate:	☐☐☐☐☐☐☐☐☐☐☐
	Target:	

Today I am proud that I: _____

_____

_____

Today I noticed that eating more and exercising less—smarter—
had a positive impact on my life when: _____

_____

_____

_____

What I ate today: _____
_____
_____
_____
_____
_____
_____
_____
_____
_____
_____

What did I do well? _____
_____
_____
_____
_____
_____
_____
_____
_____
_____
_____

Tomorrow I can eat more—smarter—5% more effectively by:
_____
_____
_____
_____
_____
_____
_____
_____
_____

Week 10—Day 3   Date:

Non-Starchy Vegetables	Ate:	☐☐☐☐☐☐☐☐☐☐
	Target:	■■■■■■■■■■
Seafood/Lean Meat/Egg Whites/Whey/Select Dairy	Ate:	☐☐☐☐☐☐☐☐☐☐
	Target:	■■■■■
Flax Seeds/Nuts	Ate:	☐☐☐☐☐☐☐☐☐☐
	Target:	■■■■■
Berries/Citrus Fruits	Ate:	☐☐☐☐☐☐☐☐☐☐
	Target:	■■■■■
Legumes	Ate:	☐☐☐☐☐☐☐☐☐☐
	Target:	
Other Fruits	Ate:	☐☐☐☐☐☐☐☐☐☐
	Target:	
Most Dairy	Ate:	☐☐☐☐☐☐☐☐☐☐
	Target:	
Fatty Meat/Oils	Ate:	☐☐☐☐☐☐☐☐☐☐
	Target:	
Starchy Vegetables/Starch	Ate:	☐☐☐☐☐☐☐☐☐☐
	Target:	
Sweets/Sweetened Drinks	Ate:	☐☐☐☐☐☐☐☐☐☐
	Target:	

Today I am proud that I: _____

_____

_____

Today I noticed that eating more and exercising less—smarter—
had a positive impact on my life when: _____

_____

_____

_____

What I ate today: _____

_____

_____

_____

_____

_____

_____

_____

_____

_____

What did I do well? _____

_____

_____

_____

_____

_____

_____

_____

_____

_____

_____

Tomorrow I can eat more—smarter—5% more effectively by:

_____

_____

_____

_____

_____

_____

_____

_____

_____

Week 10—Day 4   Date:

Non-Starchy Vegetables	Ate:	☐☐☐☐☐☐☐☐☐☐☐
	Target:	■■■■■■■■■■
Seafood/Lean Meat/Egg Whites/Whey/Select Dairy	Ate:	☐☐☐☐☐☐☐☐☐☐☐
	Target:	■■■■■
Flax Seeds/Nuts	Ate:	☐☐☐☐☐☐☐☐☐☐☐
	Target:	■■■■■
Berries/Citrus Fruits	Ate:	☐☐☐☐☐☐☐☐☐☐☐
	Target:	■■■■■
Legumes	Ate:	☐☐☐☐☐☐☐☐☐☐☐
	Target:	
Other Fruits	Ate:	☐☐☐☐☐☐☐☐☐☐☐
	Target:	
Most Dairy	Ate:	☐☐☐☐☐☐☐☐☐☐☐
	Target:	
Fatty Meat/Oils	Ate:	☐☐☐☐☐☐☐☐☐☐☐
	Target:	
Starchy Vegetables/Starch	Ate:	☐☐☐☐☐☐☐☐☐☐☐
	Target:	
Sweets/Sweetened Drinks	Ate:	☐☐☐☐☐☐☐☐☐☐☐
	Target:	

Today I am proud that I: _____

_____

_____

Today I noticed that eating more and exercising less—smarter—
had a positive impact on my life when: _____

_____

_____

_____

What I ate today: _____
_____
_____
_____
_____
_____
_____
_____
_____
_____

What did I do well? _____
_____
_____
_____
_____
_____
_____
_____
_____
_____

Tomorrow I can eat more—smarter—5% more effectively by:
_____
_____
_____
_____
_____
_____
_____
_____
_____

Week 10—Day 5   Date:

Non-Starchy Vegetables	Ate:	☐☐☐☐☐☐☐☐☐☐☐
	Target:	■■■■■■■■■■■
Seafood/Lean Meat/Egg Whites/Whey/Select Dairy	Ate:	☐☐☐☐☐☐☐☐☐☐☐
	Target:	■■■■■
Flax Seeds/Nuts	Ate:	☐☐☐☐☐☐☐☐☐☐☐
	Target:	■■■■■
Berries/Citrus Fruits	Ate:	☐☐☐☐☐☐☐☐☐☐☐
	Target:	■■■■■
Legumes	Ate:	☐☐☐☐☐☐☐☐☐☐☐
	Target:	
Other Fruits	Ate:	☐☐☐☐☐☐☐☐☐☐☐
	Target:	
Most Dairy	Ate:	☐☐☐☐☐☐☐☐☐☐☐
	Target:	
Fatty Meat/Oils	Ate:	☐☐☐☐☐☐☐☐☐☐☐
	Target:	
Starchy Vegetables/Starch	Ate:	☐☐☐☐☐☐☐☐☐☐☐
	Target:	
Sweets/Sweetened Drinks	Ate:	☐☐☐☐☐☐☐☐☐☐☐
	Target:	

Today I am proud that I: _____

_____

_____

Today I noticed that eating more and exercising less—smarter—
had a positive impact on my life when: _____

_____

_____

_____

What I ate today: _____

_____

_____

_____

_____

_____

_____

_____

_____

_____

What did I do well? _____

_____

_____

_____

_____

_____

_____

_____

_____

_____

Tomorrow I can eat more—smarter—5% more effectively by:

_____

_____

_____

_____

_____

_____

_____

_____

_____

Week 10—Day 6   Date:

Non-Starchy Vegetables
Ate: ☐☐☐☐☐☐☐☐☐☐☐
Target: ■■■■■■■■■

Seafood/Lean Meat/Egg Whites/Whey/Select Dairy
Ate: ☐☐☐☐☐☐☐☐☐☐☐
Target: ■■■■■

Flax Seeds/Nuts
Ate: ☐☐☐☐☐☐☐☐☐☐☐
Target: ■■■■■

Berries/Citrus Fruits
Ate: ☐☐☐☐☐☐☐☐☐☐☐
Target: ■■■■■

Legumes
Ate: ☐☐☐☐☐☐☐☐☐☐☐
Target:

Other Fruits
Ate: ☐☐☐☐☐☐☐☐☐☐☐
Target:

Most Dairy
Ate: ☐☐☐☐☐☐☐☐☐☐☐
Target:

Fatty Meat/Oils
Ate: ☐☐☐☐☐☐☐☐☐☐☐
Target:

Starchy Vegetables/Starch
Ate: ☐☐☐☐☐☐☐☐☐☐☐
Target:

Sweets/Sweetened Drinks
Ate: ☐☐☐☐☐☐☐☐☐☐☐
Target:

Today I am proud that I: _____
_____
_____

Today I noticed that eating more and exercising less—smarter—had a positive impact on my life when: _____
_____
_____
_____

What I ate today: _____

_____

_____

_____

_____

_____

_____

_____

_____

_____

What did I do well? _____

_____

_____

_____

_____

_____

_____

_____

_____

_____

Tomorrow I can eat more—smarter—5% more effectively by:

_____

_____

_____

_____

_____

_____

_____

_____

_____

Week 10—Day 7   Date:

		Count
Non-Starchy Vegetables	Ate:	☐☐☐☐☐☐☐☐☐☐☐
	Target:	■■■■■■■■■■
Seafood/Lean Meat/Egg Whites/Whey/Select Dairy	Ate:	☐☐☐☐☐☐☐☐☐☐☐
	Target:	■■■■■
Flax Seeds/Nuts	Ate:	☐☐☐☐☐☐☐☐☐☐☐
	Target:	■■■■■
Berries/Citrus Fruits	Ate:	☐☐☐☐☐☐☐☐☐☐☐
	Target:	■■■■■
Legumes	Ate:	☐☐☐☐☐☐☐☐☐☐
	Target:	
Other Fruits	Ate:	☐☐☐☐☐☐☐☐☐☐
	Target:	
Most Dairy	Ate:	☐☐☐☐☐☐☐☐☐☐
	Target:	
Fatty Meat/Oils	Ate:	☐☐☐☐☐☐☐☐☐☐
	Target:	
Starchy Vegetables/Starch	Ate:	☐☐☐☐☐☐☐☐☐☐
	Target:	
Sweets/Sweetened Drinks	Ate:	☐☐☐☐☐☐☐☐☐☐
	Target:	

Today I am proud that I: _____

_____

_____

Today I noticed that eating more and exercising less—smarter—
had a positive impact on my life when: _____

_____

_____

_____

What I ate today: _____

_____

_____

_____

_____

_____

_____

_____

_____

_____

What did I do well? _____

_____

_____

_____

_____

_____

_____

_____

_____

_____

Tomorrow I can eat more—smarter—5% more effectively by:

_____

_____

_____

_____

_____

_____

_____

_____

_____

Week 10 Eccentric Exercise   Date:

Home Option

		Add resistance?
Assisted Eccentric Squats	Resistance: _____	Y / N
Assisted Eccentric Pull-Ups	Resistance: _____	Y / N
Assisted Eccentric Push-Ups	Resistance: _____	Y / N
Assisted Eccentric Shoulder Press	Resistance: _____	Y / N

Gym Option

		Add resistance?
Eccentric Leg Presses	Resistance: _____	Y / N
Eccentric Rows	Resistance: _____	Y / N
Eccentric Check Presses	Resistance: _____	Y / N
Eccentric Shoulder Presses	Resistance: _____	Y / N

Week 1 Cardiovascular Exercise   Date:

		Add resistance?
10 Minutes of High-Quality Brief Cardiovascular Exercise	Resistance: _____	Y / N

Remember: It should be impossible to do more than six repetitions of each eccentric exercise per week. It should also be impossible to do more than six repetitions of brief cardiovascular exercise per week. If more repetitions are possible or more workouts are possible, then add resistance.

Notes: _____

_____
_____
_____
_____
_____
_____
_____
_____
_____

What did I do well? _____

_____
_____
_____
_____
_____
_____
_____
_____
_____

Next week I can exercise less—smarter—5% more effectively by:

_____
_____
_____
_____
_____
_____
_____
_____
_____

Week 11—Day 1   Date:

Non-Starchy Vegetables	Ate:	☐☐☐☐☐☐☐☐☐☐☐
	Target:	■■■■■■■■■■
Seafood/Lean Meat/Egg Whites/Whey/Select Dairy	Ate:	☐☐☐☐☐☐☐☐☐☐☐
	Target:	■■■■■
Flax Seeds/Nuts	Ate:	☐☐☐☐☐☐☐☐☐☐☐
	Target:	■■■■■
Berries/Citrus Fruits	Ate:	☐☐☐☐☐☐☐☐☐☐☐
	Target:	■■■■■
Legumes	Ate:	☐☐☐☐☐☐☐☐☐☐☐
	Target:	
Other Fruits	Ate:	☐☐☐☐☐☐☐☐☐☐☐
	Target:	
Most Dairy	Ate:	☐☐☐☐☐☐☐☐☐☐☐
	Target:	
Fatty Meat/Oils	Ate:	☐☐☐☐☐☐☐☐☐☐☐
	Target:	
Starchy Vegetables/Starch	Ate:	☐☐☐☐☐☐☐☐☐☐☐
	Target:	
Sweets/Sweetened Drinks	Ate:	☐☐☐☐☐☐☐☐☐☐☐
	Target:	

Today I am proud that I: _____

_____

_____

Today I noticed that eating more and exercising less—smarter—
had a positive impact on my life when: _____

_____

_____

_____

What I ate today: _____
_____
_____
_____
_____
_____
_____
_____
_____
_____

What did I do well? _____
_____
_____
_____
_____
_____
_____
_____
_____
_____

Tomorrow I can eat more—smarter—5% more effectively by:
_____
_____
_____
_____
_____
_____
_____
_____
_____

Week 11—Day 2   Date:

Non-Starchy Vegetables
Ate: □□□□□□□□□□□
Target: ■■■■■■■■■■■

Seafood/Lean Meat/Egg Whites/Whey/Select Dairy
Ate: □□□□□□□□□□□
Target: ■■■■■

Flax Seeds/Nuts
Ate: □□□□□□□□□□□
Target: ■■■■■

Berries/Citrus Fruits
Ate: □□□□□□□□□□□
Target: ■■■■■

Legumes
Ate: □□□□□□□□□□□
Target:

Other Fruits
Ate: □□□□□□□□□□□
Target:

Most Dairy
Ate: □□□□□□□□□□□
Target:

Fatty Meat/Oils
Ate: □□□□□□□□□□□
Target:

Starchy Vegetables/Starch
Ate: □□□□□□□□□□□
Target:

Sweets/Sweetened Drinks
Ate: □□□□□□□□□□□
Target:

Today I am proud that I: _____

_____

_____

Today I noticed that eating more and exercising less—smarter—had a positive impact on my life when: _____

_____

_____

_____

What I ate today: _____
_____
_____
_____
_____
_____
_____
_____
_____
_____

What did I do well? _____
_____
_____
_____
_____
_____
_____
_____
_____
_____

Tomorrow I can eat more—smarter—5% more effectively by:
_____
_____
_____
_____
_____
_____
_____
_____
_____

Week 11—Day 3   Date:

Non-Starchy Vegetables	Ate:	☐☐☐☐☐☐☐☐☐☐☐
	Target:	■■■■■■■■■■
Seafood/Lean Meat/Egg Whites/Whey/Select Dairy	Ate:	☐☐☐☐☐☐☐☐☐☐☐
	Target:	■■■■■
Flax Seeds/Nuts	Ate:	☐☐☐☐☐☐☐☐☐☐☐
	Target:	■■■■■
Berries/Citrus Fruits	Ate:	☐☐☐☐☐☐☐☐☐☐☐
	Target:	■■■■■
Legumes	Ate:	☐☐☐☐☐☐☐☐☐☐☐
	Target:	
Other Fruits	Ate:	☐☐☐☐☐☐☐☐☐☐☐
	Target:	
Most Dairy	Ate:	☐☐☐☐☐☐☐☐☐☐☐
	Target:	
Fatty Meat/Oils	Ate:	☐☐☐☐☐☐☐☐☐☐☐
	Target:	
Starchy Vegetables/Starch	Ate:	☐☐☐☐☐☐☐☐☐☐☐
	Target:	
Sweets/Sweetened Drinks	Ate:	☐☐☐☐☐☐☐☐☐☐☐
	Target:	

Today I am proud that I: _____

_____

_____

Today I noticed that eating more and exercising less—smarter—
had a positive impact on my life when: _____

_____

_____

_____

❧ THE SMARTER SCIENCE OF SLIM JOURNAL ❧

What I ate today: _____
_____
_____
_____
_____
_____
_____
_____
_____
_____
_____

What did I do well? _____
_____
_____
_____
_____
_____
_____
_____
_____
_____
_____

Tomorrow I can eat more—smarter—5% more effectively by:
_____
_____
_____
_____
_____
_____
_____
_____
_____
_____

171

Week 11—Day 4   Date:

Non-Starchy Vegetables
Ate: ☐☐☐☐☐☐☐☐☐☐☐
Target: ■■■■■■■■■■

Seafood/Lean Meat/Egg Whites/Whey/Select Dairy
Ate: ☐☐☐☐☐☐☐☐☐☐☐
Target: ■■■■■

Flax Seeds/Nuts
Ate: ☐☐☐☐☐☐☐☐☐☐☐
Target: ■■■■■

Berries/Citrus Fruits
Ate: ☐☐☐☐☐☐☐☐☐☐☐
Target: ■■■■■

Legumes
Ate: ☐☐☐☐☐☐☐☐☐☐☐
Target:

Other Fruits
Ate: ☐☐☐☐☐☐☐☐☐☐☐
Target:

Most Dairy
Ate: ☐☐☐☐☐☐☐☐☐☐☐
Target:

Fatty Meat/Oils
Ate: ☐☐☐☐☐☐☐☐☐☐☐
Target:

Starchy Vegetables/Starch
Ate: ☐☐☐☐☐☐☐☐☐☐☐
Target:

Sweets/Sweetened Drinks
Ate: ☐☐☐☐☐☐☐☐☐☐☐
Target:

Today I am proud that I: _____

_____

_____

Today I noticed that eating more and exercising less—smarter—
had a positive impact on my life when: _____

_____

_____

_____

What I ate today: _____
_____
_____
_____
_____
_____
_____
_____
_____
_____

What did I do well? _____
_____
_____
_____
_____
_____
_____
_____
_____
_____

Tomorrow I can eat more—smarter—5% more effectively by:
_____
_____
_____
_____
_____
_____
_____
_____
_____

Week 11—Day 5   Date:

Non-Starchy Vegetables	Ate:	☐☐☐☐☐☐☐☐☐☐☐
	Target:	■■■■■■■■■■
Seafood/Lean Meat/Egg Whites/Whey/Select Dairy	Ate:	☐☐☐☐☐☐☐☐☐☐☐
	Target:	■■■■■
Flax Seeds/Nuts	Ate:	☐☐☐☐☐☐☐☐☐☐☐
	Target:	■■■■■
Berries/Citrus Fruits	Ate:	☐☐☐☐☐☐☐☐☐☐☐
	Target:	■■■■■
Legumes	Ate:	☐☐☐☐☐☐☐☐☐☐☐
	Target:	
Other Fruits	Ate:	☐☐☐☐☐☐☐☐☐☐☐
	Target:	
Most Dairy	Ate:	☐☐☐☐☐☐☐☐☐☐☐
	Target:	
Fatty Meat/Oils	Ate:	☐☐☐☐☐☐☐☐☐☐☐
	Target:	
Starchy Vegetables/Starch	Ate:	☐☐☐☐☐☐☐☐☐☐☐
	Target:	
Sweets/Sweetened Drinks	Ate:	☐☐☐☐☐☐☐☐☐☐☐
	Target:	

Today I am proud that I: _____

_____

_____

Today I noticed that eating more and exercising less—smarter—
had a positive impact on my life when: _____

_____

_____

_____

What I ate today: _____

_____

_____

_____

_____

_____

_____

_____

_____

_____

What did I do well? _____

_____

_____

_____

_____

_____

_____

_____

_____

_____

Tomorrow I can eat more—smarter—5% more effectively by:

_____

_____

_____

_____

_____

_____

_____

_____

_____

Week 11—Day 6   Date:

Non-Starchy Vegetables	Ate:	☐☐☐☐☐☐☐☐☐☐
	Target:	■■■■■■■■■■
Seafood/Lean Meat/Egg Whites/Whey/Select Dairy	Ate:	☐☐☐☐☐☐☐☐☐☐
	Target:	■■■■■
Flax Seeds/Nuts	Ate:	☐☐☐☐☐☐☐☐☐☐
	Target:	■■■■■
Berries/Citrus Fruits	Ate:	☐☐☐☐☐☐☐☐☐☐
	Target:	■■■■■
Legumes	Ate:	☐☐☐☐☐☐☐☐☐☐
	Target:	
Other Fruits	Ate:	☐☐☐☐☐☐☐☐☐☐
	Target:	
Most Dairy	Ate:	☐☐☐☐☐☐☐☐☐☐
	Target:	
Fatty Meat/Oils	Ate:	☐☐☐☐☐☐☐☐☐☐
	Target:	
Starchy Vegetables/Starch	Ate:	☐☐☐☐☐☐☐☐☐☐
	Target:	
Sweets/Sweetened Drinks	Ate:	☐☐☐☐☐☐☐☐☐☐
	Target:	

Today I am proud that I: _____

_____

_____

Today I noticed that eating more and exercising less—smarter—
had a positive impact on my life when: _____

_____

_____

_____

What I ate today: _____

_____

_____

_____

_____

_____

_____

_____

_____

_____

What did I do well? _____

_____

_____

_____

_____

_____

_____

_____

_____

_____

Tomorrow I can eat more—smarter—5% more effectively by:

_____

_____

_____

_____

_____

_____

_____

_____

Week 11—Day 7   Date:

Non-Starchy Vegetables	Ate:	☐☐☐☐☐☐☐☐☐☐☐☐
	Target:	■■■■■■■■■■
Seafood/Lean Meat/Egg Whites/Whey/Select Dairy	Ate:	☐☐☐☐☐☐☐☐☐☐☐
	Target:	■■■■■
Flax Seeds/Nuts	Ate:	☐☐☐☐☐☐☐☐☐☐☐
	Target:	■■■■■
Berries/Citrus Fruits	Ate:	☐☐☐☐☐☐☐☐☐☐☐
	Target:	■■■■■
Legumes	Ate:	☐☐☐☐☐☐☐☐☐☐☐
	Target:	
Other Fruits	Ate:	☐☐☐☐☐☐☐☐☐☐☐
	Target:	
Most Dairy	Ate:	☐☐☐☐☐☐☐☐☐☐☐
	Target:	
Fatty Meat/Oils	Ate:	☐☐☐☐☐☐☐☐☐☐☐
	Target:	
Starchy Vegetables/Starch	Ate:	☐☐☐☐☐☐☐☐☐☐☐
	Target:	
Sweets/Sweetened Drinks	Ate:	☐☐☐☐☐☐☐☐☐☐☐
	Target:	

Today I am proud that I: _____

_____

_____

Today I noticed that eating more and exercising less—smarter—
had a positive impact on my life when: _____

_____

_____

_____

What I ate today: _____

_____

_____

_____

_____

_____

_____

_____

_____

_____

What did I do well? _____

_____

_____

_____

_____

_____

_____

_____

_____

_____

_____

Tomorrow I can eat more—smarter—5% more effectively by:

_____

_____

_____

_____

_____

_____

_____

_____

_____

Week 11 Eccentric Exercise   Date:

Home Option

		Add resistance?
Assisted Eccentric Squats	Resistance: _____	Y / N
Assisted Eccentric Pull-Ups	Resistance: _____	Y / N
Assisted Eccentric Push-Ups	Resistance: _____	Y / N
Assisted Eccentric Shoulder Press	Resistance: _____	Y / N

Gym Option

		Add resistance?
Eccentric Leg Presses	Resistance: _____	Y / N
Eccentric Rows	Resistance: _____	Y / N
Eccentric Check Presses	Resistance: _____	Y / N
Eccentric Shoulder Presses	Resistance: _____	Y / N

Week 1 Cardiovascular Exercise   Date:

		Add resistance?
10 Minutes of High-Quality Brief Cardiovascular Exercise	Resistance: _____	Y / N

Remember: It should be impossible to do more than six repetitions of each eccentric exercise per week. It should also be impossible to do more than six repetitions of brief cardiovascular exercise per week. If more repetitions are possible or more workouts are possible, then add resistance.

Notes: _____

_____

_____

_____

_____

_____

_____

_____

_____

_____

_____

What did I do well? _____

_____

_____

_____

_____

_____

_____

_____

_____

_____

_____

Next week I can exercise less—smarter—5% more effectively by:

_____

_____

_____

_____

_____

_____

_____

_____

_____

_____

Week 12—Day 1   Date:

Non-Starchy Vegetables	Ate:	☐☐☐☐☐☐☐☐☐☐☐☐
	Target:	■■■■■■■■■■
Seafood/Lean Meat/Egg Whites/Whey/Select Dairy	Ate:	☐☐☐☐☐☐☐☐☐☐☐☐
	Target:	■■■■■
Flax Seeds/Nuts	Ate:	☐☐☐☐☐☐☐☐☐☐☐☐
	Target:	■■■■■
Berries/Citrus Fruits	Ate:	☐☐☐☐☐☐☐☐☐☐☐☐
	Target:	■■■■■
Legumes	Ate:	☐☐☐☐☐☐☐☐☐☐☐☐
	Target:	
Other Fruits	Ate:	☐☐☐☐☐☐☐☐☐☐☐☐
	Target:	
Most Dairy	Ate:	☐☐☐☐☐☐☐☐☐☐☐☐
	Target:	
Fatty Meat/Oils	Ate:	☐☐☐☐☐☐☐☐☐☐☐☐
	Target:	
Starchy Vegetables/Starch	Ate:	☐☐☐☐☐☐☐☐☐☐☐☐
	Target:	
Sweets/Sweetened Drinks	Ate:	☐☐☐☐☐☐☐☐☐☐☐☐
	Target:	

Today I am proud that I: _____

_____

_____

Today I noticed that eating more and exercising less—smarter—
had a positive impact on my life when: _____

_____

_____

_____

What I ate today: _____

_____

_____

_____

_____

_____

_____

_____

_____

_____

What did I do well? _____

_____

_____

_____

_____

_____

_____

_____

_____

_____

_____

Tomorrow I can eat more—smarter—5% more effectively by:

_____

_____

_____

_____

_____

_____

_____

_____

_____

Week 12—Day 2   Date:

Non-Starchy Vegetables	Ate:	☐☐☐☐☐☐☐☐☐☐
	Target:	■■■■■■■■■■
Seafood/Lean Meat/Egg Whites/Whey/Select Dairy	Ate:	☐☐☐☐☐☐☐☐☐☐
	Target:	■■■■■
Flax Seeds/Nuts	Ate:	☐☐☐☐☐☐☐☐☐☐
	Target:	■■■■■
Berries/Citrus Fruits	Ate:	☐☐☐☐☐☐☐☐☐☐
	Target:	■■■■■
Legumes	Ate:	☐☐☐☐☐☐☐☐☐☐
	Target:	
Other Fruits	Ate:	☐☐☐☐☐☐☐☐☐☐
	Target:	
Most Dairy	Ate:	☐☐☐☐☐☐☐☐☐☐
	Target:	
Fatty Meat/Oils	Ate:	☐☐☐☐☐☐☐☐☐☐
	Target:	
Starchy Vegetables/Starch	Ate:	☐☐☐☐☐☐☐☐☐☐
	Target:	
Sweets/Sweetened Drinks	Ate:	☐☐☐☐☐☐☐☐☐☐
	Target:	

Today I am proud that I: _____

_____

_____

Today I noticed that eating more and exercising less—smarter—had a positive impact on my life when: _____

_____

_____

_____

What I ate today: _____

_____

_____

_____

_____

_____

_____

_____

_____

_____

What did I do well? _____

_____

_____

_____

_____

_____

_____

_____

_____

_____

Tomorrow I can eat more—smarter—5% more effectively by:

_____

_____

_____

_____

_____

_____

_____

_____

_____

Week 12—Day 3   Date:

Non-Starchy Vegetables	Ate:	☐☐☐☐☐☐☐☐☐☐
	Target:	■■■■■■■■■■
Seafood/Lean Meat/Egg Whites/Whey/Select Dairy	Ate:	☐☐☐☐☐☐☐☐☐☐
	Target:	■■■■■
Flax Seeds/Nuts	Ate:	☐☐☐☐☐☐☐☐☐☐
	Target:	■■■■■
Berries/Citrus Fruits	Ate:	☐☐☐☐☐☐☐☐☐☐
	Target:	■■■■■
Legumes	Ate:	☐☐☐☐☐☐☐☐☐☐
	Target:	
Other Fruits	Ate:	☐☐☐☐☐☐☐☐☐☐
	Target:	
Most Dairy	Ate:	☐☐☐☐☐☐☐☐☐☐
	Target:	
Fatty Meat/Oils	Ate:	☐☐☐☐☐☐☐☐☐☐
	Target:	
Starchy Vegetables/Starch	Ate:	☐☐☐☐☐☐☐☐☐☐
	Target:	
Sweets/Sweetened Drinks	Ate:	☐☐☐☐☐☐☐☐☐☐
	Target:	

Today I am proud that I: _____

_____

_____

Today I noticed that eating more and exercising less—smarter—
had a positive impact on my life when: _____

_____

_____

_____

What I ate today: _____
_____
_____
_____
_____
_____
_____
_____
_____
_____

What did I do well? _____
_____
_____
_____
_____
_____
_____
_____
_____
_____

Tomorrow I can eat more—smarter—5% more effectively by:
_____
_____
_____
_____
_____
_____
_____
_____
_____

Week 12—Day 4   Date:

		Ate:	Target:
Non-Starchy Vegetables	Ate:	□□□□□□□□□□□	
	Target:	■■■■■■■■■■	
Seafood/Lean Meat/Egg Whites/Whey/Select Dairy	Ate:	□□□□□□□□□□□	
	Target:	■■■■■	
Flax Seeds/Nuts	Ate:	□□□□□□□□□□□	
	Target:	■■■■■	
Berries/Citrus Fruits	Ate:	□□□□□□□□□□□	
	Target:	■■■■■	
Legumes	Ate:	□□□□□□□□□□□	
	Target:		
Other Fruits	Ate:	□□□□□□□□□□□	
	Target:		
Most Dairy	Ate:	□□□□□□□□□□□	
	Target:		
Fatty Meat/Oils	Ate:	□□□□□□□□□□□	
	Target:		
Starchy Vegetables/Starch	Ate:	□□□□□□□□□□□	
	Target:		
Sweets/Sweetened Drinks	Ate:	□□□□□□□□□□□	
	Target:		

Today I am proud that I: _____

_____

_____

Today I noticed that eating more and exercising less—smarter—
had a positive impact on my life when: _____

_____

_____

_____

What I ate today: _____

_____

_____

_____

_____

_____

_____

_____

_____

_____

What did I do well? _____

_____

_____

_____

_____

_____

_____

_____

_____

_____

Tomorrow I can eat more—smarter—5% more effectively by:

_____

_____

_____

_____

_____

_____

_____

_____

_____

Week 12—Day 5   Date:

Non-Starchy Vegetables	Ate:	☐☐☐☐☐☐☐☐☐☐☐
	Target:	■■■■■■■■■■
Seafood/Lean Meat/Egg Whites/Whey/Select Dairy	Ate:	☐☐☐☐☐☐☐☐☐☐☐
	Target:	■■■■■
Flax Seeds/Nuts	Ate:	☐☐☐☐☐☐☐☐☐☐☐
	Target:	■■■■■
Berries/Citrus Fruits	Ate:	☐☐☐☐☐☐☐☐☐☐☐
	Target:	■■■■■
Legumes	Ate:	☐☐☐☐☐☐☐☐☐☐☐
	Target:	
Other Fruits	Ate:	☐☐☐☐☐☐☐☐☐☐☐
	Target:	
Most Dairy	Ate:	☐☐☐☐☐☐☐☐☐☐☐
	Target:	
Fatty Meat/Oils	Ate:	☐☐☐☐☐☐☐☐☐☐☐
	Target:	
Starchy Vegetables/Starch	Ate:	☐☐☐☐☐☐☐☐☐☐☐
	Target:	
Sweets/Sweetened Drinks	Ate:	☐☐☐☐☐☐☐☐☐☐☐
	Target:	

Today I am proud that I: _____

_____

_____

Today I noticed that eating more and exercising less—smarter—
had a positive impact on my life when: _____

_____

_____

_____

What I ate today: _____
_____
_____
_____
_____
_____
_____
_____
_____
_____

What did I do well? _____
_____
_____
_____
_____
_____
_____
_____
_____
_____
_____

Tomorrow I can eat more—smarter—5% more effectively by:
_____
_____
_____
_____
_____
_____
_____
_____
_____
_____

Week 12—Day 6   Date:

Non-Starchy Vegetables	Ate:	☐☐☐☐☐☐☐☐☐☐☐	
	Target:	■■■■■■■■■■	
Seafood/Lean Meat/Egg Whites/Whey/Select Dairy	Ate:	☐☐☐☐☐☐☐☐☐☐☐	
	Target:	■■■■■	
Flax Seeds/Nuts	Ate:	☐☐☐☐☐☐☐☐☐☐☐	
	Target:	■■■■■	
Berries/Citrus Fruits	Ate:	☐☐☐☐☐☐☐☐☐☐☐	
	Target:	■■■■■	
Legumes	Ate:	☐☐☐☐☐☐☐☐☐☐☐	
	Target:		
Other Fruits	Ate:	☐☐☐☐☐☐☐☐☐☐☐	
	Target:		
Most Dairy	Ate:	☐☐☐☐☐☐☐☐☐☐☐	
	Target:		
Fatty Meat/Oils	Ate:	☐☐☐☐☐☐☐☐☐☐☐	
	Target:		
Starchy Vegetables/Starch	Ate:	☐☐☐☐☐☐☐☐☐☐☐	
	Target:		
Sweets/Sweetened Drinks	Ate:	☐☐☐☐☐☐☐☐☐☐☐	
	Target:		

Today I am proud that I: _____

_____

_____

Today I noticed that eating more and exercising less—smarter—
had a positive impact on my life when: _____

_____

_____

_____

What I ate today: _____

_____

_____

_____

_____

_____

_____

_____

_____

What did I do well? _____

_____

_____

_____

_____

_____

_____

_____

_____

Tomorrow I can eat more—smarter—5% more effectively by:

_____

_____

_____

_____

_____

_____

_____

_____

Week 12—Day 7   Date:

Non-Starchy Vegetables	Ate:	☐☐☐☐☐☐☐☐☐☐☐
	Target:	■■■■■■■■■■
Seafood/Lean Meat/Egg Whites/Whey/Select Dairy	Ate:	☐☐☐☐☐☐☐☐☐☐☐
	Target:	■■■■■
Flax Seeds/Nuts	Ate:	☐☐☐☐☐☐☐☐☐☐☐
	Target:	■■■■■
Berries/Citrus Fruits	Ate:	☐☐☐☐☐☐☐☐☐☐☐
	Target:	■■■■■
Legumes	Ate:	☐☐☐☐☐☐☐☐☐☐☐
	Target:	
Other Fruits	Ate:	☐☐☐☐☐☐☐☐☐☐☐
	Target:	
Most Dairy	Ate:	☐☐☐☐☐☐☐☐☐☐☐
	Target:	
Fatty Meat/Oils	Ate:	☐☐☐☐☐☐☐☐☐☐☐
	Target:	
Starchy Vegetables/Starch	Ate:	☐☐☐☐☐☐☐☐☐☐☐
	Target:	
Sweets/Sweetened Drinks	Ate:	☐☐☐☐☐☐☐☐☐☐☐
	Target:	

Today I am proud that I: _____

_____

_____

Today I noticed that eating more and exercising less—smarter—
had a positive impact on my life when: _____

_____

_____

_____

What I ate today: _____

_____

_____

_____

_____

_____

_____

_____

_____

_____

What did I do well? _____

_____

_____

_____

_____

_____

_____

_____

_____

_____

Tomorrow I can eat more—smarter—5% more effectively by:

_____

_____

_____

_____

_____

_____

_____

_____

_____

Week 12 Eccentric Exercise   Date:

Home Option

		Add resistance?
Assisted Eccentric Squats	Resistance: _____	Y / N
Assisted Eccentric Pull-Ups	Resistance: _____	Y / N
Assisted Eccentric Push-Ups	Resistance: _____	Y / N
Assisted Eccentric Shoulder Press	Resistance: _____	Y / N

Gym Option

		Add resistance?
Eccentric Leg Presses	Resistance: _____	Y / N
Eccentric Rows	Resistance: _____	Y / N
Eccentric Check Presses	Resistance: _____	Y / N
Eccentric Shoulder Presses	Resistance: _____	Y / N

Week 1 Cardiovascular Exercise   Date:

		Add resistance?
10 Minutes of High-Quality Brief Cardiovascular Exercise	Resistance: _____	Y / N

Remember: It should be impossible to do more than six repetitions of each eccentric exercise per week. It should also be impossible to do more than six repetitions of brief cardiovascular exercise per week. If more repetitions are possible or more workouts are possible, then add resistance.

Notes: _____

_____

_____

_____

_____

_____

_____

_____

_____

_____

What did I do well? _____

_____

_____

_____

_____

_____

_____

_____

_____

_____

Next week I can exercise less—smarter—5% more effectively by:

_____

_____

_____

_____

_____

_____

_____

_____

_____

CPSIA information can be obtained at www.ICGtesting.com
Printed in the USA
BVOW062223170612

292929BV00002B/1/P